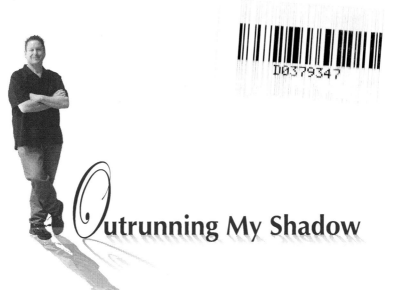

Outrunning My Shadow

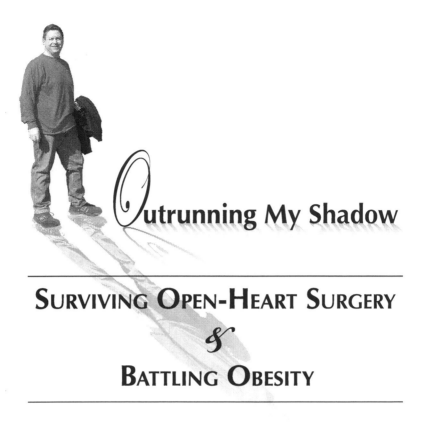

Outrunning My Shadow

SURVIVING OPEN-HEART SURGERY

&

BATTLING OBESITY

The Decision to Change My Life

KEITH AHRENS

Foreword by Dr. Eric Wikler

To order additional copies, please contact us:

www.outrunningmyshadow.com

keith@outrunningmyshadow.com

Nihoa Press

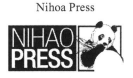

www.NihoaPress.com

Cover Design / Book Design / Illustration / Production: Amy Ahrens Gureckis

Photography: Susan Lipman, Carla Stephens, Peter Duveen,
Nicole Fay, Jimmy Lee, Chelsea Arce, Family & Friends

Dedicated to the memory of my mother and guardian angel.

Thanks for inspiring and teaching me.

You would be so proud.

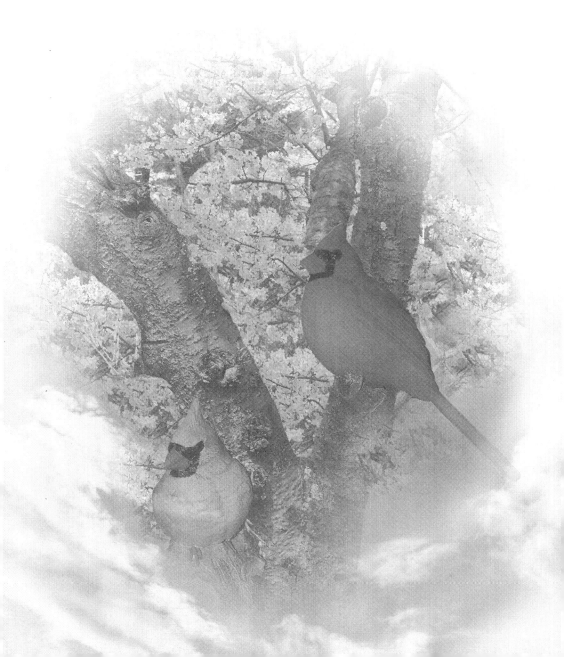

Keith, you of all people should know what it's like to value life and to be able to live life to the fullest. Take the opportunity now to follow your dreams. The last thing you want is to regret not following your dreams while the opportunity is there.

Lynn

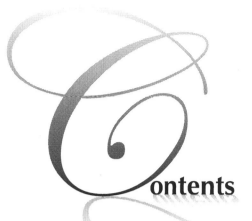

ontents

*Nothing will ever be attempted
if all possible objections must first be overcome*

Samuel Johnson

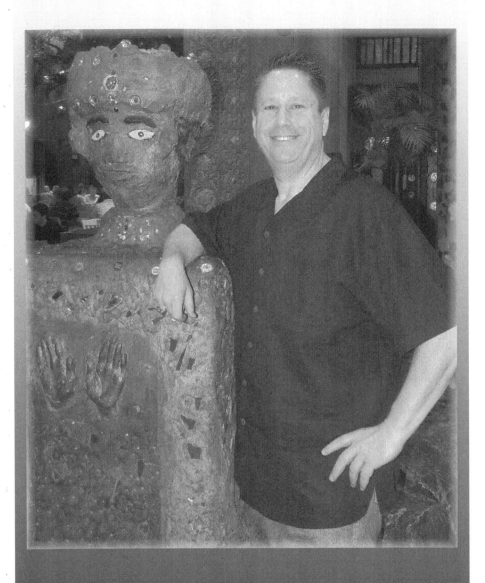

Giving to others was the greatest gift I ever received

Keith Ahrens
Author, Outrunning My Shadow

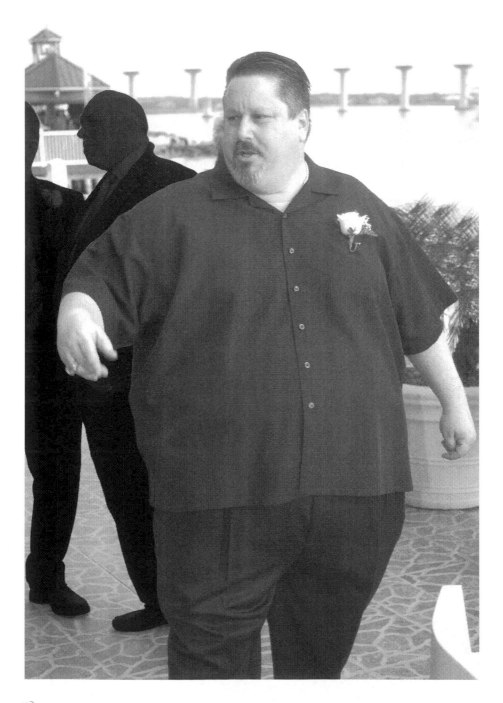

Foreword

by Dr. Eric Wikler, D.O.

Keith walked into my office in April 2007 having no idea that he had just made the first step in a journey that would forever change his life. As Keith was pacing the exam room, clearly in extreme distress, he informed me that he had not been feeling well and had experienced several episodes of dizziness and fatigue. He had not had a physical in over ten years, weighed over 400 pounds, and was very concerned for his health. Even though he had waited so long, time was now of the essence. I ordered a full panel of blood work and performed an EKG, and to my surprise his labs only revealed a slight elevation in his cholesterol. However, Keith's EKG had an abnormality that ultimately revealed that he had had a heart attack.

Unfortunately, in family practice this is not an unusual occurrence. Many patients wait until they have symptoms before they visit the doctor instead of having regular exams to screen for risk factors. The difference in Keith's case is the resulting remarkable journey that he has taken. Keith has been an inspiration to me, other health care providers, and his family and friends. He has achieved the single greatest weight loss I have seen through what I consider the "right way," good old-fashioned diet and exercise.

Obesity is an epidemic in our country. Approximately 60% of Americans are either overweight or obese. The United States is one of the most advanced nations in the world in science and medicine; however, we are ranked number 32 in lifespan. What is the cause of this dichotomy? My feeling is that obesity has become a side effect of the American way of life. Proper diet and exercise are followed by very few Americans. We work long hours, have hectic busy lives, and find ourselves with little time for much else. When we do have those precious free moments, the last thing on our minds is exercising. Therefore, it is a challenge for nearly everyone to overcome the obstacles to fitness.

In my experience, I have found there are three main groups of dieters and exercisers. Group One is the non-active group. These are the people that are not exercising and not watching their diet. They may be thinking about it or wishing that they were thinner, but they are not taking any action. I often see these patients in my office, and they tend to comment that they cannot seem to lose the weight, but when I question them, they either have not made an attempt or they have tried and failed and given up.

Group Two is either dieting and/or exercising; however, they are inconsistent; they experience limited success with weight loss and tend to regain weight easily. Although this group is better than Group One, they are not reaching their goals and still leave themselves at increased health risk.

Group Three is actively exercising regularly, and dieting is a way of life for them, not just a short- term program. This group is definitely in the minority, though it is the group that we should all strive to be in. Most people tend to be in Group Two, but we do move in and out of these groups at different times in our lives. It is the job of the family practitioner to identify which group an individual is in and encourage him or her to improve and stay motivated.

If a person adheres to a sensible diet and includes the appropriate level of exercise, he or she will lose weight. It's that simple. The main problem people have with diets is that they go on them until they have either given up or lost the weight, and then they return to their old eating habits, and subsequently their weight rebounds. In my opinion, the best diet is a diet that never stops. This means that we need to make better, healthier food choices. Weight loss will occur more easily if we choose to eat more fish, chicken, fruits, vegetables, salads (with healthy dressing), less fast food, and fewer fatty meats and heavy carbohydrates. With healthier lifestyle choices, all of us can be in Group Three!

Though critically important to a healthy lifestyle, diet is only half the battle. Exercise is equally important, not just for weight loss but for improving heart health. Ideally, one should exercise continuously for 45 to 60 minutes at his/her target heart rate at least five days per week. I recommend starting off slow, even if the patient can only last five minutes. If the workout can be increased just a few minutes each time, the patient will quickly reach his or her goal. Picking an exercise that the patient enjoys—or at least somewhat enjoys—is essential. It doesn't matter if it's running, biking, walking, the elliptical, or the stepper. Exercise will burn calories and increase the metabolism, causing continued calorie loss throughout the day. As long as the target heart rate can be reached and kept there, weight will be lost and kept off.

In addition to the benefits of weight loss, exercise also improves circulation to the heart. When the heart pumps the blood, the first place the blood goes is back to the heart through the coronary arteries, providing oxygen to the cardiac muscle. A heart attack (myocardial infarction) occurs when plaque ruptures from the lining of the coronary artery and travels downstream until it lodges in the artery and blocks the blood flow. The area downstream of the blockage does not receive oxygenated blood and subsequently dies. Exercise develops increased collateral circulation. The heart is a muscle that when exercised is pumping harder and requires more oxygen. The body achieves this increase in oxygen by growing new blood vessels that supply the heart with its increased demand. When a heart attack occurs, an exercising individual will have less damage than his or her sedentary counterpart due to these very important collaterals. As such, routine exercise will burn calories, reduce weight, and improve heart health.

Diet and exercise are the cornerstones to our longevity. There are many variables to an individual's life span, yet only a few are under our control. I have seen seemingly healthy patients with no risk factors have heart attacks at a young age. I have also seen overweight smokers and heavy drinkers live into their eighties. Genetics obviously has a major role in our health, and though we cannot do anything about the hand that we are dealt, we can play it to the best of our ability. In general, a person who exercises regularly, follows a healthy diet, drinks no more than one to two alcoholic beverages a day, avoids cigarettes, and controls blood pressure, cholesterol, and blood sugars will maximize his or her health and feel the benefits on a daily basis.

It took a crisis for the light to go on for Keith. He is now an amazing champion in the fight for fitness, and I admire his drive and determination. Over the last two years, I have found myself looking forward to his office visits for the inspiration he continues to instill in me. At a recent office visit, Keith told me about this book and shared with me that he wanted people to take the initiative toward good health and visit their physicians for a checkup. Simply establishing a baseline will allow a physician to screen a patient for health risk factors that may ultimately prevent life threatening diseases such as cardiovascular disease.

I hope that people will be inspired by Keith's story and become advocates for their own health and well-being. I encourage patients to take responsibility for their health, to get in the driver's seat, and to see where the journey takes them.

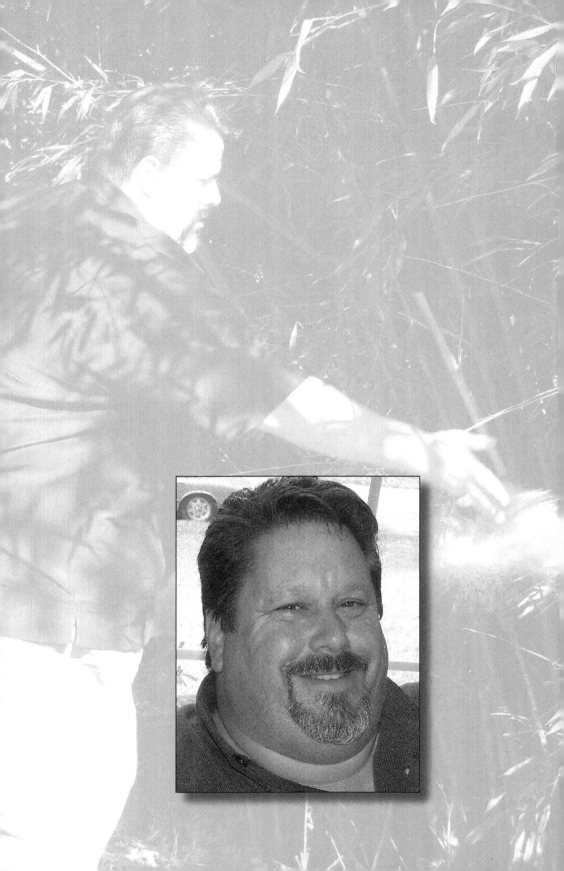

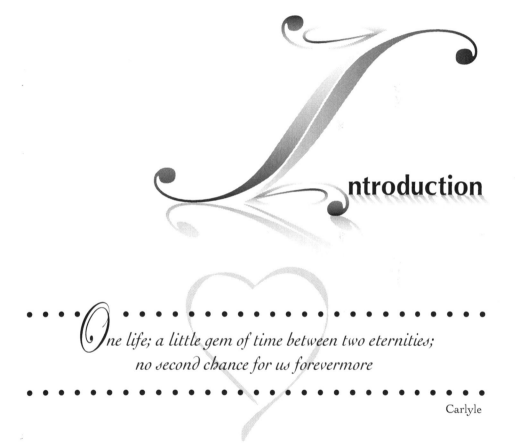

Introduction

*One life; a little gem of time between two eternities;
no second chance for us forevermore*

Carlyle

I never thought that I would get an opportunity or, quite frankly, have the desire to write a book about some recent experiences that have changed my life. I feel that by sharing my story I can reach out and help someone else who may be facing the same or similar problems or trying to prevent them. I hope to inspire you or someone you know to take control and make a difference in your lives for better physical fitness and health.

This book is not just about a fat guy who got sick and lost a bunch of weight. It is much more. It's about a journey that we all hope to take in life that leads us to a better place. The journey never stops. We hope it only gets better. No matter where we start, at whatever age, we can improve our situation no matter how bad the odds seem stacked against us. It is amazing what we can do when we put our minds to it. Every day we read in the paper or see on television or hear our friends tell us about this or that person who did something so great we can hardly believe it. What we all have to understand is that *we* are those people. We have it in ourselves to do something great.

If a friend asks us about our greatest dream, we may tell him or her that winning the lottery would be the greatest thing. Sure, money would be great, but someone told me a long time ago that "If money can fix it, it really isn't a problem." When you are faced with a health issue or you have a friend or loved one that is sick, you don't often think about money. Our health is the one thing we can't take for granted. There are so many things we can do to create a healthier life. Very few things in any health-related prevention situation are not in our control. The main one that is out of our control is our genetics. You know the old saying, "You can choose your friends, but you can't choose your family." Family history of medical problems and genetics plays such a key role in so many health problems we may face. Understanding that, we can change the things we can control and take control of the things we can't change.

I have had a great life. I grew up in suburban Maryland just outside of Washington D.C. I was one of seven children, four sisters and two brothers. I was the youngest of three boys and had two older and two younger sisters. I had a great mother who always encouraged me and was always proud of my accomplishments. I loved my mother more than anything in the world.

My parents divorced when I was thirteen. My dad was a successful businessman and remarried a kind and decent woman. Growing up, I lived with my mom. I went to college and began working right out of college and never looked back. I have only had a few jobs since leaving college. I ran a retail division for a large office products company. I taught an aerospace engineering project with my cousin Charles. We worked with learning disabled and deaf children and with inner city minority students, and we also trained teachers who were working on advanced graduate credits. I have worked in the automobile business for the past 14 years. When I look back, I can honestly say that I loved all of the jobs I had, but I think I liked teaching the best.

I did not have the best eating habits while I was growing up, and they spiraled out of control when I went out on my own. Mom never had salt and pepper on the table, and on the rare occasion they were on the table, if we put salt or pepper on our food before taking the first bite, we were going to be in trouble. Needless to say, I never had a sodium problem. I ate a lot of fried foods and foods with high fat content. I loved fast foods. I ate a lot of crap and had terrible eating habits. I am definitely a compulsive overeater. I often ate after I was full and often ate when I wasn't even hungry. I just loved food and felt so good when I ate. I ate so often out of emotion and very often by myself.

The people I was around every day had no idea how much I would eat or binge on late at night. I remember so many times feeling completely out of control with my eating habits. It is something I will struggle with the rest of my life. Being aware of this problem has been the foundation for my ongoing recovery. I was athletic when I was younger, but after graduating college and going to work I led a very sedentary lifestyle.

I was recently diagnosed at the young age of only 45 with having had a Remote Silent Heart Attack. Subsequently, I underwent open-heart coronary artery bypass surgery. I have also lost over ***185 pounds*** by making healthier food choices and exercising regularly. Perhaps this story will inspire you or a loved one to encourage, support, and coach someone you care about to better health. Maybe we have a friend that can use our support. We all have to remember that "What happens to us, happens to our family and friends." Any illness that happens to us, or a goal we are trying to reach, affects not just ourselves but the people around us. I had heart surgery and have lost a lot of weight by eating right and exercising regularly.

It is this

story that I

want to share . . .

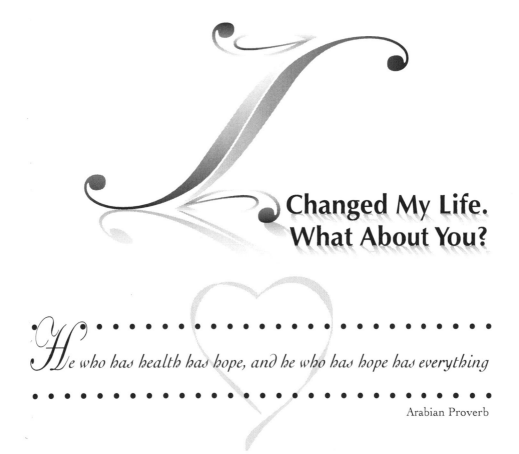

Changed My Life. What About You?

He who has health has hope, and he who has hope has everything

Arabian Proverb

What would it take for you to make a decision to change your life?

Looking at your kids without a parent?

Looking at your parents without a kid?

Looking at your spouse without you?

Looking at your brothers and sisters without you?

Not being able to share your life with close friends?

We are all faced with so many personal and professional problems every day. Family issues seem to always be pressing us to the limit. Whatever our daily problems are, we need to step back and look in the mirror. If we don't have our health, we can't help others, much less ourselves.

I know that the decision to change one's life should start with getting a checkup. Each of us should know what hand we are holding. I have encouraged many of my friends and people I have met to just go see a doctor for a physical. I believe that just knowing where you stand is better than the unknown. If the only thing you do after reading this book, or even if you stop reading here, is make an appointment with your doctor for a checkup, I feel I have done my part.

For me, the decision to change my life was learning that I might have a heart problem and my acute awareness of my obesity and how it affected my quality of life. I knew that if I didn't change my life dramatically, I would die sooner than I wanted to. It really hit home for me the day of my stress test and my first cardiologist visit with Dr. Spaccavento on May 23, 2007. I thought that if by chance the tests he was going to put me through showed anything at all, I had better start getting myself in better shape.

I used to joke with my co-workers that if I died, everyone would say the same things at my funeral. They would say, "Boy, he was always at work," "He sure worked hard," "He was a hard worker," and "Keith never took time off for himself." I didn't want to die sitting at my desk and completely out of shape. I wanted to live. I knew I had to do something now and it could not wait.

I not only had to get physically fit and start to eat right, but I had to lose a lot of weight. I thought about how many people cared about me and loved me. I thought about not wanting to leave them. I just wasn't ready to give up. I didn't want to let anyone down, but I also knew I had to do this for myself. It was finally time I took matters into my own hands. I knew I had to set short-term and long-term realistic goals that I could track to literally see my achievement. I felt I had just gotten a slight advantage in the fact that I had just seen the doctor and I knew what my baseline medical numbers were. I had my checkup, and knew where I stood. I knew I would get the support and encouragement of my family and friends. There have been many times that I feel I am on an island by myself. I know that the choices I make are mine. I realized a long time ago that no one could do it for me.

I

now had

to be

in control . . .

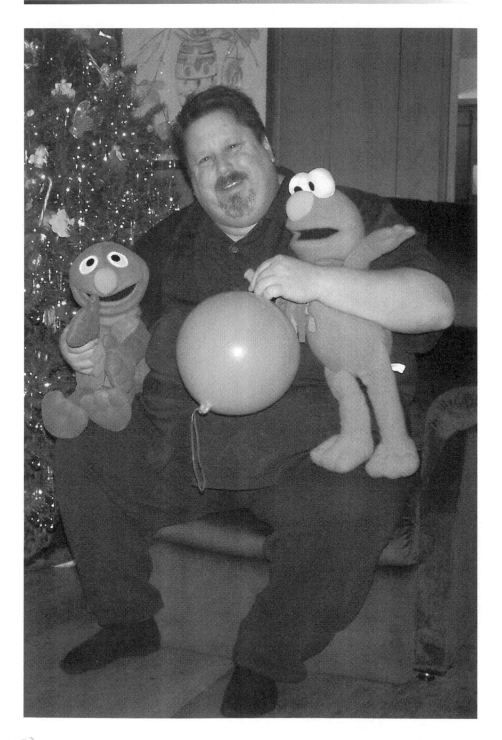

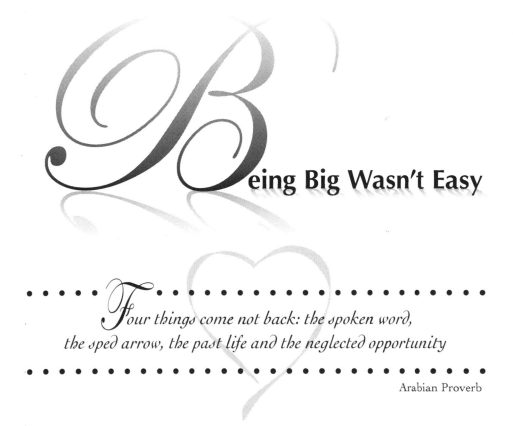Being Big Wasn't Easy

*Four things come not back: the spoken word,
the sped arrow, the past life and the neglected opportunity*

Arabian Proverb

Being a big person is difficult, to say the least. It is easy to think that a fat person is making a choice to be fat. It is easy to think that fat people just don't care about themselves but could control the urge to eat whenever they wanted. The same is often said about a smoker, alcoholic, or drug addict. I once told someone that I was glad that I was not an alcoholic or drug addict because with my compulsive eating behavior, I would probably be dead. After I said that, I quickly realized that I was in fact killing myself and was going to die from my overeating. I am not making excuses or trying to convince someone that some of us can't control what we do; rather, I'm telling the story of making the decision for yourself, within yourself, that you are going to change the things you can now. When you are obese, people look at you differently and treat you differently.

I was talking with one of my best friends one day. He happens to be an African American. We were having a conversation and the subject of race came up and how many people can't understand what it is like to be black in America from a discrimination standpoint in certain situations. I made the comment that I don't know any more about being a black person in America than someone thin knows what it's like to be walking around in a 400-plus pound body.

Discrimination comes in all shapes, colors, and—in my case—sizes. There are so many situations when people pass judgment on the overweight person. Sometimes getting a table at a restaurant was difficult. You always wondered how the hostess or host was looking at you. You wondered where they would seat you. I got used to that and always requested a table that I was happy with. I often thought that everyone in the restaurant was looking at me to see how much I ate. I always needed a chair without arms. I could never sit in a booth. No matter what I ordered, I thought I was ordering too much and often did. Just ordering one item on the menu was a challenge. I always made it a double when I could. It seemed like it was a race to eat as much as I could every time I ate.

Flying on an airplane was brutal. I used to buy two seats or pay for first class when I could afford it. I always needed a seatbelt extender. I hated to ask the flight attendant for it. God forbid you had to go to the bathroom or the lavatory as they call it on an airplane. Look how small the doors are and then how small the area is once inside. It was frightening. I always prayed I would not have to go to the bathroom on an airplane.

When I took my nieces or nephews to an amusement ride, I felt so bad that I couldn't go on the ride with them. I remember being with a niece and nephew and getting to the front of the line for an amusement park ride, and when I tried to get seated with them, I could not put the safety bar down in front of me. I had to get off the ride and wait for them.

The list goes on. I used to wait a long time at the shopping center or wherever I was going for a parking space up front because I had difficulty walking because I was in such bad shape. At work I always needed a chair with no arms and one that seemed a little sturdier than the rest. I remember everyone getting new furniture at work, and I had to make a case for myself to keep my old, unsightly chair because of the way it felt. I knew it wasn't going to break underneath me. Going to an outdoor event or place where they used those cheap un-sturdy chairs was frightening. I remember wondering if the chair could even hold me. I remember trying to think of what excuse to use, although so obvious, if the chair broke. I had to sit sideways on a picnic bench because I could not fit at the table. When I would go to dinner with a friend at a mall that involved a few minutes' walk, I would have to stop and pretend I was looking in the store windows just to catch my breath. If I had someone with me at work,

I would always try to drive. I knew that by going in their car it was going to be hard for me to get in and out. Sitting in the passenger seat was a pain in the neck. I remember always being so uncomfortable. Often in my case the seatbelt never fit. I had a friend that wanted to take me on a helicopter ride once. I could not get the seatbelt around me and had to get off. When I went to a stadium to see a sporting event, I could not fit in the seats. I would have to sit on the front edge of the seat because the sides were too narrow. There are so many examples of the struggles one would face when being so obese. These were just a few of the daily obstacles I faced. The actual list is much longer.

I have dieted on and off my entire adult life. I have gained and lost more weight than anyone can imagine. I guess the problem was that I was dieting and not making the proper lifestyle changes to support my weight loss. The pounds always came back on, and then some. I hate the word *dieting*. I think of the word as an "overused excuse to fall back on your old eating habits." Think about it. What happens when you are not dieting? You are clearly going back to your old, un-healthy ways. I believe now that for success to occur long-term, you have to accept that the changes you make now, whether it be eating healthier or exercise or both, are forever. That is the way it is. If we learn to accept that, we can succeed. I struggle every day, and I am reminded everyday when I look in the mirror of how I used to be.

Maybe I needed to love the new me

more than the old me?

$\mathcal{M}$y Story

Health is achieved by gaining awareness of that area of life from where the totality of life can be easily handled. The total potential of life lies in the field of pure awareness which offers infinite creativity and all possibilities

Maharishi Mahesh Yogi

It was the first week in April, 2007. I was 45 years old, 5'10" tall, and weighed at least 414 pounds. The reason I say at least 414 pounds is that when I visited my doctor for the first time, he did not have a scale that would go over 400 pounds. I was first accurately weighed at my first visit to the cardiologist office on May 23, 2007. In recent years, as far as physical exertion and movement, I was not in good shape at all. Doing the simplest things, such as walking to the car or climbing a flight of stairs, was a chore. Heavy breathing and shortness of breath always followed. I remember walking up the two short flights of stairs separated by a landing to our business office at work and stopping to catch my breath before going into the office so that no one would see me breathing hard. They probably knew that I was trying to hide it. I did the same for our sales meetings. When no one was behind me, I would stand just outside the door to the conference room to catch my breath. I used to walk up the stairs to my bedroom and be so out of breath.

There were times when I had such severe heartburn. I took antacid tablets and never thought that it could be artery blockage that was causing such discomfort. When you are obese, you always blame any warning signs of potential heart disease on the fact that you are just fat. I never put into perspective that I could be developing or had developed a serious medical problem. I worked a lot of hours every day in a high stress environment, but I loved my work. Up until the last few years I was always able to move fast for a big man. I always projected that I had a lot of energy. I think that my outgoing personality made me seem much more energetic to co-workers and friends than I actually was.

One night in the first week of April, I was lying at the foot of my bed watching television before going to sleep. I sat up and got extremely lightheaded. I sat on the edge of the bed for a few minutes and thought I had just gotten up too quickly. I had not had that feeling before and thought it was very strange. After a few minutes and taking a few deep breaths, the lightheadedness went away and I went to sleep.

A couple of days later, I had another episode, but it was a little more severe. I remembered a slight feeling of nausea and more intense dizziness. I was able to regain my composure and chalked that up to just not eating right or whatever excuse I thought of that moment. Another couple days went by and I was at my desk at work, casually talking to Allen, one of my co-workers. He was sitting across from me. I was talking with him and looking down at my computer. As we were talking, I lifted my head from my computer and remembered getting very lightheaded. I felt real nauseous. I remember looking straight at him and not hearing a word he was saying. It was a very bizarre moment. He kept talking, but I couldn't hear him. I was getting dizzier, and I was just thinking to myself, *Keith, you don't want to pass out here.* I started breathing slowly just trying to clear my head and regain my composure. He did not have a clue I was not feeling well.

He got up and left my office and then another one of my co-workers came in to the office. His name was Allen also, and I told him I wasn't feeling very well, and I asked him if he could go get my car and pull it around to the side of the building that was a lot closer to my office. I honestly thought that if I had to walk to my car on the other side of the lot I could not make it without passing out. I thought that if I could just sit back in my car seat, I would feel better. He pulled my car up outside my office and again I told him I wasn't feeling too good and would probably just go home and relax and lie down. He knew something wasn't quite right with me because I never, ever left work and hardly ever took time off if I were sick. I was able to get to my car and I just sat in it for what seemed like hours. He checked up on me knowing something wasn't right. I told him I would be fine and that I just needed to relax a bit. I could see out of the corner of my eye that he never took his eyes off me.

To be honest, just sitting in the car seat felt good. I felt like all of my energy had been sapped out of me. I was there for about 30-45 minutes, just sitting there breathing slowly, trying to relax. I felt so tired. When he checked up on me again, I told him I was going home to lie down for a couple of hours. He wanted to drive me home, but I assured him I was fine. I ended up driving myself home and going straight to bed. I fell asleep almost immediately.

When I woke up a few hours later, and thank God I woke up, I knew that I needed to go see a doctor and get checked out. I needed a physical. I needed a checkup. I had not had one in about 10 years since my sister Stacy passed away from leukemia. You would have thought that my sister Stacy's passing would have been a wake up call for a better lifestyle. It is truly amazing what may motivate an individual to wake up and take action. When I woke up, I called Allen at work as I promised him I would and told him I was fine and not to worry. I remember telling him I was just so tired and knew a good nap was all that I needed.

It was later diagnosed that these episodes of dizziness, shallow breathing, fatigue, and slight nausea were most likely happening as a result of what the doctors call a Remote Silent Heart Attack. I should have been in the hospital. I never knew I had one, but it was later diagnosed this way. The warning signs were so clear that I was having a heart-related problem. I should have headed right for the hospital instead of getting in my car and going home to go to sleep. I was very lucky to be alive. By being single and living by myself, I wouldn't have been able to yell and hope someone would come if I fell ill.

It is so important

to understand

the warning

signs of a

possible

heart attack...

and seek

immediate medical attention!

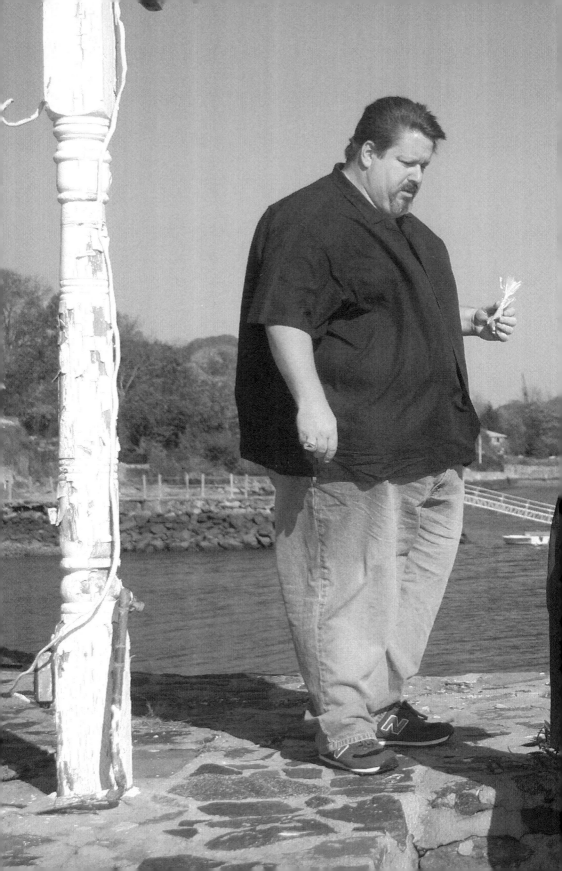

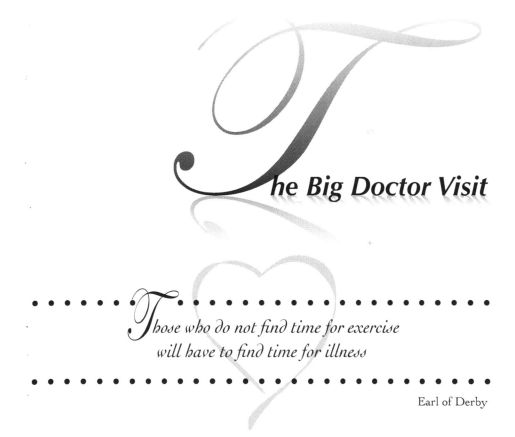

The Big Doctor Visit

*Those who do not find time for exercise
will have to find time for illness*

Earl of Derby

A couple of days later, I got the name of a family doctor from our controller, Nikki. The doctor's name was Eric Wikler. I scheduled the appointment and went in for my first visit. I think that when he saw me, he was thinking, *This guy is huge and out of shape*, and from the way I described what was going on, I think he was thinking that I had diabetes or something like that.

My blood pressure was good and I didn't have any more dizzy spells after that first week. I thought I was going to be fine and that he would just tell me to lose weight and exercise. He wanted me to schedule a complete physical at which time we would go over my blood work, and so on. I took his lab orders, and I went to get all my blood work done and scheduled my physical with him a week later. I liked this doctor from the first time I met him. He took his time to listen to me, and he asked a lot of questions. He was sincere and told me that his focus after we found out what was wrong with me would always be on prevention and taking care of myself.

When I returned to his office for my complete physical, I remember his being a little surprised that my blood sugar check for diabetes was normal. My cholesterol and triglycerides were elevated, but I didn't know at the time what these numbers all meant. He did a prostate exam, my first. That appeared to be normal. Even my cancer screening came back OK. As part of a routine physical, he did an EKG, or electrocardiogram, to look at my heart rhythm. After everything was done, he came in the office and sat down.

He told me that aside from having to lose weight and exercise, which I knew he would say, an abnormality or something showed up on my EKG and that he wanted to get a heart stress test administered by a cardiologist. He didn't want to leave any stone unturned. He told me that the machines they used to monitor the heart in a doctor's office for routine physicals are not nearly as advanced as a machine that a cardiologist or hospital would use. He even told me that it may be nothing at all but wanted to make sure, and he also said that a stress test at my age would be a good thing since I had not had one in nearly ten years. He referred me to a cardiologist and the stress test was scheduled. Dr. Wikler knew how to treat the high, bad cholesterol and the low, good cholesterol and my triglyceride level.

Thank God

that this doctor

had the experience

and knowledge

to take me

to the next level.

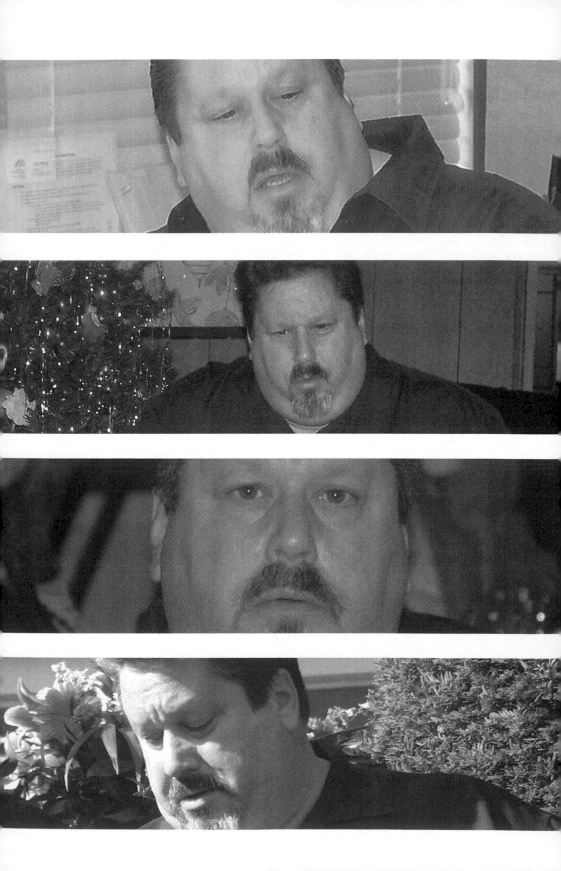

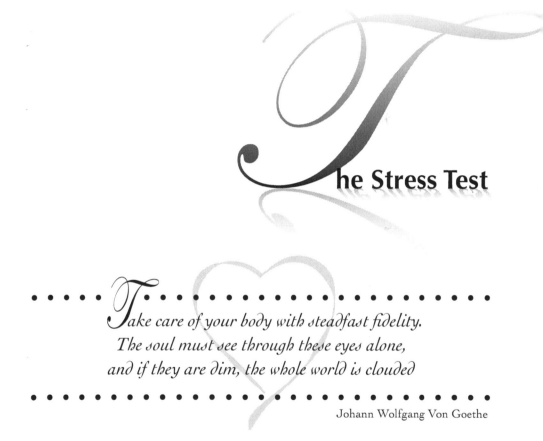

The Stress Test

Take care of your body with steadfast fidelity.
The soul must see through these eyes alone,
and if they are dim, the whole world is clouded

Johann Wolfgang Von Goethe

Stress tests are normally done in a cardiologist's office, but due to my large size and weight, the cardiologist said they needed to do it at a local hospital. They call it a nuclear stress test because during the stress test they administer what I presume is a nuclear "dye" and take slow, steady pictures of the heart to see if there is any shading which may indicate arterial blockage or other possible problems.

The tests appear as high resolution pictures of the heart and show up in different color images to reveal open or blocked arterial passages. If I had to describe the machine they use to take the images, I would say that it is like an MRI scanner. The normal procedure is that they inject the patient with the nuclear material and then they take images of the heart. After the initial images, the stress test is administered. This test is normally done on a treadmill but can also be done in a different way if the person can't walk or get on a treadmill due to mobility or physical limitations.

Let's stick to the treadmill for now. The nurse or doctor gets you on the treadmill and gets you going. The idea is to get the heart rate up to a certain percentage of the maximum heart rate to see if there are any abnormalities. They will get the heart rate up in a hurry no matter what shape a patient is in. Keep in mind that the patient is hooked up to an electrocardiogram machine and a blood pressure monitor the whole time so that they can monitor the heart.

About halfway through the stress test, they administered another dose of the nuclear medicine. After finishing the stress test, the patient goes back to the imaging scanner for another set of pictures. I assume that before and after shots are necessary to see the arteries at rest and at exertion stages to determine potential blockages.

There is no pain at all in the stress test. The only problem I had was a severe anxiety attack when I got to the hospital. I was thinking that

I had no family with me at the time: I was by myself. If something went wrong, no one would be there to help me. When the nurses took my blood pressure before the test, it was off the charts. I mean it was really off the charts. I have never had high blood pressure, and the nurses thought I was going to bust the machine. After I saw the concern on their faces, I told them that the reading they were getting was not correct and that their blood pressure monitor was wrong. They hooked me up to another monitor, and it was also off the chart. My anxiety level was through the roof for no reason. They actually stopped the testing on me and wanted a doctor to see me. I went across the street to the cardiologist's office to see the doctor, who saw me immediately and listened to my heart and took my blood pressure.

Everything was fine at that moment. He told me that my heart sounded good and that he thought I was a little excited about the test. He told me to relax and to get my ass back to the hospital and finish the test. I felt so much better and was really relaxed after that. I went back to the hospital and saw the cardiac nurses. They took my blood pressure and wanted to know what the doctor had given me to make my blood pressure normal. I told them he had given me nothing and that it was just anxiety and that I was totally relaxed now. They were OK with that, and we completed the test.

There are a couple of details here that I should add. The cardiologist wrote a note to the cardiac nurse to not have me do the treadmill but rather the lying down stress test. Remember, earlier I said that some people can't use a treadmill to get their heart going because of certain physical limitations or mobility problems. I will try to describe the lying down stress test.

The nurse had me lie down on a bed. An IV was started. They basically inject a patient with something that I believe dilates the blood vessels in the heart to simulate physical exertion, like a treadmill would. It is a strange feeling, but again it is not painful. A good nurse will walk a patient through the test every moment and "coach" him along. I had a great nurse that kept me comfortable the whole time.

I finished the stress test and even got a chance to see my images on the monitor before the doctor could interpret them. I was scheduled to see the cardiologist a few days later.

The images

looked good to me,

but what the hell

did I know?

The Stress Test Results

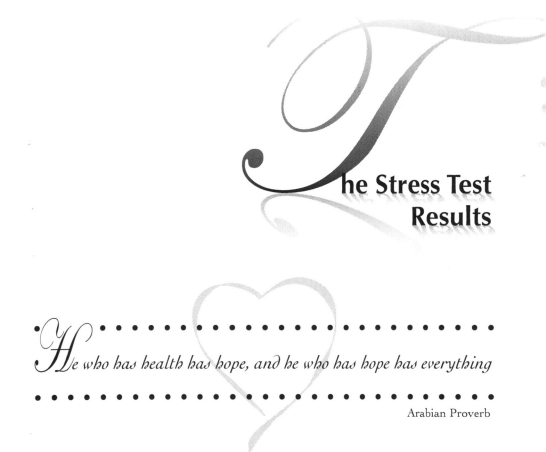

He who has health has hope, and he who has hope has everything

Arabian Proverb

I went a few days later to the cardiologist's office to get my results. Dr. Spaccavento is a board-certified cardiologist and was recommended by Dr. Wikler. I checked him out and he had a great reputation and was known as a leader in the field of cardiology in the Las Vegas area. I felt lucky that I also liked him from the first time I met him. He was up on all of the latest medical procedures and advancements in the field of cardiology. I honestly thought that everything was going to be ok and that I would be advised to lose weight and exercise. When I got there, he came into the room and told me that there was some "shading" on my stress test images and that he would like to do a more thorough test that would be totally conclusive. He told me that the accuracy in the stress test is exceptionally good, but further investigation was warranted. He then said that an angiogram procedure would provide definitive conclusions as to any blockage and, more importantly, where the blockages were and the extent of any blockages in the coronary arteries.

The angiogram procedure, also called a cardiac catheterization, is an invasive procedure done in a hospital in the catheterization lab. Normally, a catheter is inserted into the femoral artery just below the belt line where the leg meets the hip, below the stomach. The femoral artery is the main artery that goes from your heart down the leg. The catheter is then inched up through the artery near the heart. You are awake although lightly sedated during the procedure. When the catheter gets near the heart, the doctor then injects a dye that goes into the heart. It is seen on a monitor and is recorded to disk. An x-ray movie of the heart is taken when the dye is administered. The doctor is then able to see any blocked or narrowing passages of the arteries feeding the heart. A determination can then be made if any further procedure should be done. There are other angiogram procedures being done now; one that is rapidly evolving involves a non-invasive scan much like an MRI (Magnetic Resonance Imaging) or CAT Scan (CT Scan—Computerized Axial Tomography).

Your doctor would guide you as to the best course of action should one be warranted. The new technology is advancing quickly, and perhaps one day there will be no need for an invasive procedure like I had.

When he told me we needed to schedule the angiogram, he was concerned that my weight and size could be a problem for the hospital table that I would lie on when the procedure would be performed. The table is narrow and must be able to move back and forth during the procedure. As it turned out, the room was fine and the table was able to hold me. I left his office, and when I got into the car, I called my sister Candy to see if she would fly out to Las Vegas and be with me for the procedure. I didn't want another thing done without some family with me, to avoid the same high-anxiety mindset that I had for the stress test. She agreed to come out.

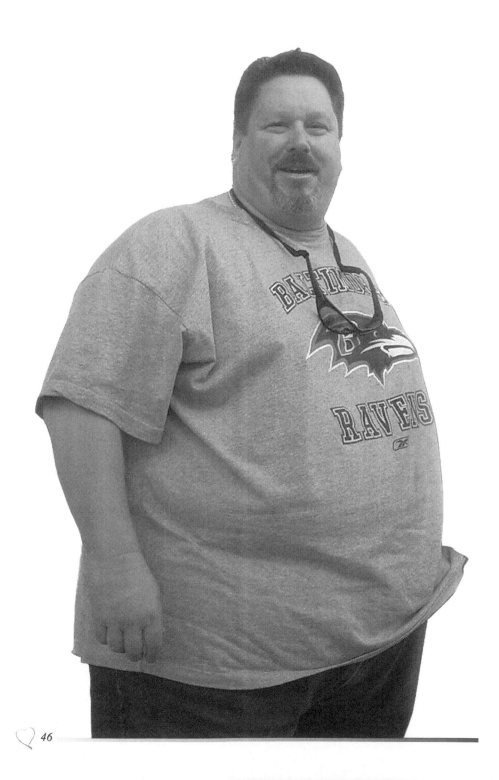

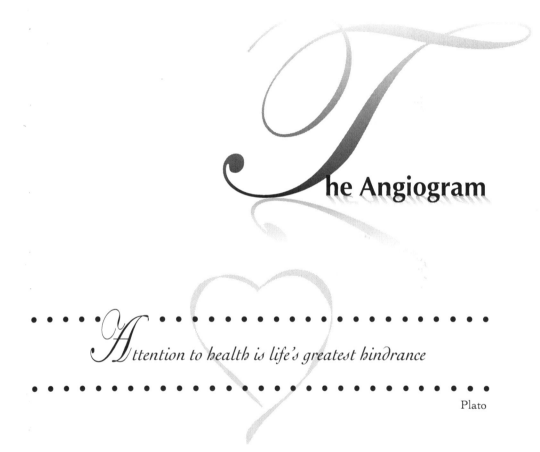

The Angiogram

Attention to health is life's greatest hindrance

Plato

It was July 6. I remembered on the night of July 5, I walked on the treadmill for about 22 minutes, which was about ¾ of a mile. I felt really good. I had been exercising for about a month and a half at this point. My weight was down that morning to 380 pounds from the 414 I started at on May 23 when I was first weighed at the cardiologist's office. I felt that I was doing all the right things. I remember going into the angiogram thinking that the worst thing that the doctor would tell me was that I would need a stent, if I needed anything at all.

From my understanding, there are four things that can happen when you go for an angiogram, depending on the percentage of blockage discovered in the arteries of the heart.

 Nothing – There is insufficient blockage to call for a procedure at that time. In some patients, however, the walls of the arteries are too weak to do a procedure. This may be the case in some very old patients.

 Angioplasty – A small balloon is inserted in the artery. Once inside the arterial wall, the balloon is inflated, thus pushing any plaque against the walls of the artery to give it a bigger opening for blood to flow.

 Stent – A small tube is put inside the artery and then it is expanded like a tunnel, allowing greater blood flow.

 Coronary Artery Bypass Surgery – Also referred to as CABG (Coronary artery bypass grafting) and commonly only as bypass surgery, this procedure involves removing a piece of a vein or artery from another location in the patient and attaching it at the location of the blocked artery to restore blood flow. Depending on the number of bypasses needed, the procedure can be labeled single, double, triple, quadruple bypass, and so on.. This procedure is performed typically if the blockage is severe or there is no blood flow at all.

When I got to the hospital for the angiogram, I put on a hospital gown and weighed in. I was then taken into another room where a nurse took all my vitals and asked a score of medical questions. I was then taken into the room where the procedure was done. The room seemed to be on the chilly side. There were at least three techs in there to get me ready for the procedure and to assist the cardiologist. They prepped me by laying me down on the table. It was a long, thin metal table.

One of the techs came over and told me he had to make sure the area was sterile and he proceeded to shave my pubic hair and the surrounding area. That was quite a feeling. Then I remember one guy checking to see where my femoral artery was. This is the main artery that goes to the heart from the leg area. It is located at the top front of the leg near the joint. When he applied pressure to the femoral artery to check for pulse and position, I actually giggled because it tickled a little bit. I believe this is the most common entry place for the catheter to the heart since it is a straight shot. It seems like a long way, but I was doing as I was told.

The doctor came in, and I remember the room being cold. I tried to zone myself out and think of being in a different place. The procedure itself was not painful to me as much as it was uncomfortable. After he put the catheter in and snaked it up to my heart, he then injected the dye. I remember a monitor that would actually allow a patient to watch the procedure as it was being done, but I just closed my eyes or looked at the ceiling.

Once the dye was injected, I remember the doctor quickly saying,

" *Keith, we have a problem;*

this is not good.

You have three

completely occluded arteries."

He then told me he was going to talk to my sister, who was in the waiting room. I remember him leaving the room, and I started to shake. I felt like I was freezing. I remember getting so cold all of a sudden. I was a little worried because I had never planned on him saying what he did, or even in my wildest imagination that my arteries would be completely blocked. I thought...

What was I to do Now?

The techs then got me ready for the recovery room by applying pressure to the artery on the outside of my leg. It was uncomfortable, but I knew I could deal with it. I then was moved to the recovery room where my sister was waiting for me. I think she had already called some of my brothers and sisters to let them know what was going on, but she didn't tell me.

After the procedure you have to lie flat for a few hours and not move your leg so that the artery can seal itself. Lying flat and not moving for a few hours is uncomfortable and irritating. I have told others that I believe it is mind over matter to lie still, and I really had to psych myself up for it. The nurses are continually checking up on you. The nurses are checking around the entry site for any type of hardness, which could indicate bleeding. I was doing as I was told by the nurses because I knew that it was the fastest way out of there.

Candy and I waited, and my cardiologist came back out to talk to us. When he arrived, he told me that I had three completely occluded (blocked) arteries. He also said that my heart had developed and grown over the years an unusually large number of collateral veins and arteries that had been feeding my heart as the blockages had gotten worse. Remember, with no blood flow to the heart, you are in a dangerous situation. He told me that this condition did not develop over the last year or two but was many years in the making, along with family genetics. He also told me that heart disease is becoming more prevalent in younger people. There were many factors that led to this point, but he told me that we must deal with what we have now. The cardiologist said that the surgeon on duty was in surgery and would come talk to me soon about my options when he finished. My cardiologist told me that I would most likely have to have surgery to correct my blockages and allow blood to flow back to the heart.

While waiting for the surgeon to come talk to me, I remember feeling really depressed. I was thinking that this is the worst possible situation I could be in.

Could there be any worse news?

I was thinking to myself that I had let myself down.

I thought I had let all of my family down.

How the hell did I get myself into this situation?

How could I have done this to myself?

I thought about all my bad eating habits over the years.

I thought how sedentary my life was for so many years.

I was wishing that I was able to turn the clock back.

After a couple of hours, the surgeon on call at the hospital came to my bedside. He told me that based on his evaluation of the angiogram results that I would need surgery to correct the blockages. He also told me that because of my weight and size that I should get down to 300 pounds before he would operate on me, to reduce the risk factors that could complicate the surgery. He felt I had a greater risk of dying during the surgery at my current weight and size. He told me I would need at least a triple bypass.

I remember asking him if exercising and losing weight could reverse and open up the blocked arteries so that I would not need surgery. He told me unequivocally "No." He said that cardiac artery bypass surgery was the only way to correct the problem. When he told me I needed to get down to 300 pounds before he could operate on me, it just didn't sound right. I mean, this guy was telling me I needed open heart surgery and to come back in four or five months *if* I could lose the weight to get it done? I could tell that this advice did not sit well with my cardiologist, who told me to come see him in his office in a few days to go over my options after I recovered from the angiogram.

I was going to leave the hospital and have to tell my employer, family, and friends that in a few months I needed open-heart surgery. This sounded crazy even to me. I remember thinking no one would ever believe me. Hell, I didn't believe it. I kept thinking that I was only 45. This isn't supposed to happen for 20 more years.

Here is a letter I emailed to a few friends and family
after the angiogram:

Hi, guys.

Let me tell you what's been going on with me over the past few weeks. We are close friends and don't want to appear to be hiding anything from you. I have not shared this with everyone, yet so please keep this private although it is not a secret and I understand everyone's genuine concerns. I am dealing with a serious health issue but believe everything will work out.

The following is a brief description of what's happening and it kind of tells the story. The following is part of a letter and info that was sent to a doctor at Johns Hopkins Hospital in Baltimore.

I had an angiogram on July 6, 2007, and was told that I had all three major arteries completely blocked and there maybe more blockage. I was told I need coronary bypass surgery but because of my weight on the 6th of 380 pounds, the cardiac surgeon on call decided that due to what I am assuming were my vital signs, he felt that I should wait until my weight got down to 300 pounds before surgery. Dr. Spaccavento, my cardiologist, told me my heart was strong and that an army of collateral veins or arteries over the years has taken over the blood and oxygen supply to my heart. I meet with Dr. Spaccavento on July 18th and will learn more from him after the hospital visit and angiogram that

I had on the 6th. In the 2 months prior to my angiogram, I had gone from 414 lbs to 380 the day of the angiogram. My blood pressure was normal and my cholesterol had come down to 149, I believe. For two months I had been eating a very low fat diet and walking on my treadmill. I had worked up to about 22 minutes at a distance of 3/4 to .8 of a mile. I felt really good. The last time I walked was the night before the angiogram. I felt I was doing all the right things.

This is my story that led up to the angiogram; about 3 months ago I got lightheaded three times in a period of one week. On a scale of 1-10, 10 being passed out, I would say I had a 6, a 7.5 and a 9. After the nine I decided to go see a doctor for a physical, which I had not had in years. It is important to note I have not had any more light headiness. I saw Dr. Eric Wikler, D.O., Wikler Family Practice 702-***-****; he ordered blood work and the results just showed high cholesterol. He prescribed Lipitor®, and I continue to take it today. All of my other stuff came back ok. He did an EKG and an abnormality showed up and he told me a stress test would be warranted. He referred me to Cardiologist Dr. Spaccavento and we did the nuclear stress test without the treadmill, i.e., me lying on my back and they gave me the IV that raced my heart. The results I believe showed signs of a possible blockage on an artery. Dr. Spaccavento then thought an angiogram was in order. At the angiogram I believe he was quite surprised to find the extent of blockage that he found.

Since I sent this letter to Hopkins, I met with the cardiologist again and am down to 370 and all my vitals are remarkably good. Blood pressure is perfect 120 over 80, my cholesterol is at 130 total 79 bad cholesterol. I feel ok at this time I am still doing all the right things. My sister Candy has been here until we sort all this out and has been a huge help. I thought she would drive me crazy but just the opposite has happened.

That's a synopsis of what's up. I am getting a 2nd opinion from the Cleveland Clinic in

Cleveland Ohio, a third opinion from Johns Hopkins in Baltimore, and a fourth opinion from another surgeon here in Vegas. This is not something that has happened over the past year or two but over my lifetime. It is not a matter of if I need the surgery but when is the big question, and where to have it done. Most people would not have left the hospital, but because of my size they decided to wait. Obviously there is much anxiety and emotions but I will be fine. The thing that is really helping me through this is that it is me and not my nieces, nephews, brothers, sisters, or my close friends that is in this situation.

I will definitely keep you posted, but I thought you should know what's up. Everything will work out fine.

Keith

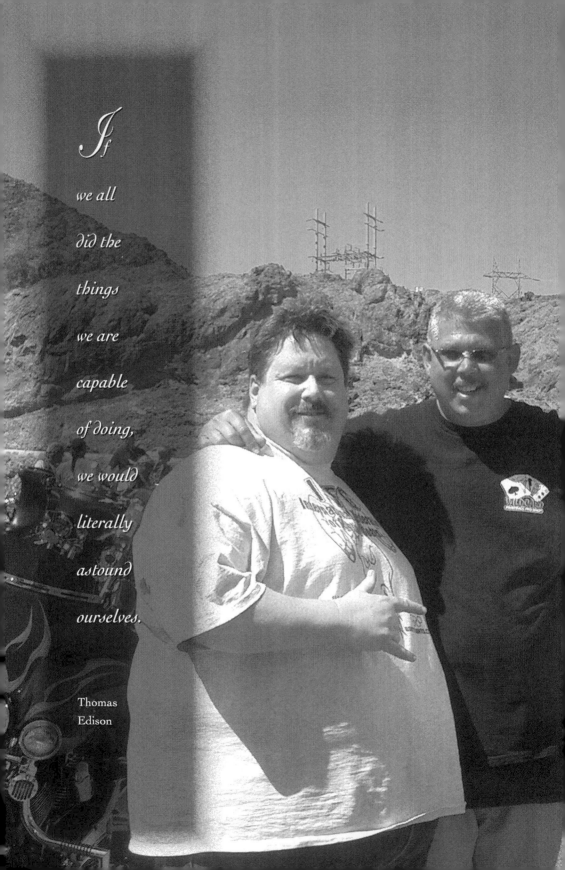

If

we all

did the

things

we are

capable

of doing,

we would

literally

astound

ourselves.

Thomas
Edison

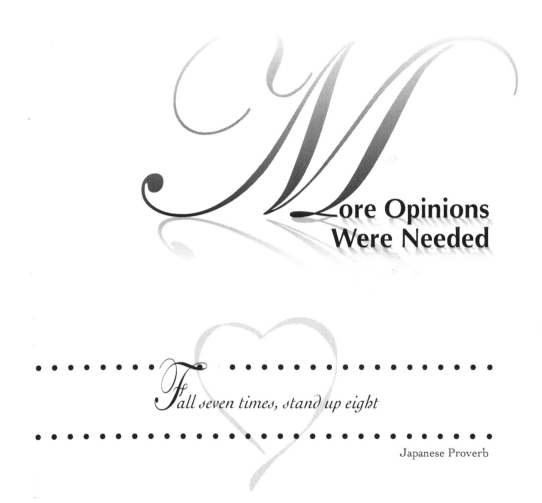

More Opinions Were Needed

Fall seven times, stand up eight

Japanese Proverb

I knew I would need more surgical and medical opinions quickly and with that in mind, the next few days I made many phone calls. My sister and I quickly researched the top heart hospitals in the United States. Hell, I was thinking that if I was going to have my chest cut open, I was going to have it done at the best hospital in the country. I remembered that my good friend Ian had a brother who I had met at his wedding ten years earlier. I remembered his brother Glen was a doctor. Not only was he a doctor, he was a cardiologist at Johns Hopkins Hospital in Baltimore, Maryland. I asked Ian if he would mind if I called his brother for some advice. I remember what Ian said to me as if it were yesterday. He said that with what I was facing that I should call in all my favors and seek whatever help I could. He told me that this was a time not to hold back anything. He said that I was always generous with my time with others and always trying to help other people and that now was the time to concentrate on me. I must add that Ian was a good guy to talk to because several years earlier he was faced with a life-changing medical issue and understood what I was going through. I was able to get hold of Dr. Glen, and he was happy to assist me and review my medical information. I quickly sent him all of my medical records for his review and opinion.

I also found out that the Cleveland Clinic, the number one rated heart hospital in the United States and possibly the world, did what is known as an e-consult. It is a second opinion or consultation done using the internet. There was a cost to this service not covered by insurance, but to have an opinion from them was going to be valuable. A lengthy medical questionnaire is filled out along with specific questions you want their team of cardiologists and surgeons to answer for you. All of my medical records were also forwarded to the Cleveland Clinic. Once they are reviewed, they issued a medical opinion. This whole process takes only a couple of weeks.

Don was another one of my close friends whom I called. His wife, Hanna, is a doctor with a cardiology background, and I spoke with her. She was very familiar with the cardiac surgeons and the coronary care units at the local hospitals. I asked her bluntly that if it were her husband and my friend Don that was faced with having open-heart surgery, who would she have do it and where would she have it done. As it turned out, the answers and recommendations she gave me were the same choices I made for my own surgeon and hospital. She encouraged me to do my research and ask as many questions as I could of the doctors or any other health care provider I was speaking with or considering.

In the meantime, Candy and I were still researching the top hospitals and cardiac departments in the Las Vegas area. We also did the research to find the top cardiac surgeons in the area and their qualifications. We checked on their board certifications along with their experience. Several names kept rising to the top of our list. Let's face it: most people when told they need to have open-heart surgery do not get a chance to leave the hospital much less do any research to select their own surgeon. The surgeon on call is normally the doctor who operates. I was lucky that I had a chance to make some of my own choices. I am sure there are many great heart surgeons out there, but I wanted the best. In researching the hospitals I also called some of the head nurses at the local hospitals. I would ask them which surgeon they would pick and where they would have the surgery if they were in my shoes. I asked a lot of questions. I got a lot of answers that needed to be sorted out and evaluated.

I went back to visit the cardiologist again, and we went over my angiogram results. He thought that I was doing all of the right things by getting more opinions. He felt I would need the surgery sooner rather than later, but he was not a surgeon. He encouraged me to speak with two of the top heart surgeons in the Las Vegas area.

I had narrowed my list to three surgeons in the area. I set appointments and interviewed two of the top surgeons on my list. Each one was board certified and had an outstanding reputation. I had a long list of questions that I posed to both of them. They each answered all of my questions. I grilled each one on my diagnosis and their prognoses for my recovery. At first I was curious about their bedside manners and friendliness, then I remembered Dr. Wikler, my primary doctor, telling me that a primary doctor should have great bedside manners and be real nice and friendly while helping you with preventive medicine and any illness you may have at the time. He said that a cardiologist should be straightforward about the heart and more matter of fact in dealing with you. He said I shouldn't care if my surgeon is friendly or not as long as he or she is a brilliant surgeon at the top of his or her game with outstanding credentials and an equally great reputation in the medical community.

I was very lucky in that I liked both of the surgeons I interviewed. Each had diagnosed me as having a Myocardial Infarction, or heart attack. Each recommended the surgery be done as soon as possible. One of the surgeons told me that I had over a 25% chance of having a non-survivable heart attack within a year without the surgery. Both of the surgeons informed me of the increased risk of death during surgery due to my weight. They both felt that they could perform the surgery with positive results despite my weight. I believe I had found the best of the best and eventually would decide on one of these surgeons.

Out of the eight total medical opinions I received from board-certified cardiologists and surgeons, only one said to wait for surgery until my weight got to down to 300 pounds. This wait could have been several months. All of the other opinions agreed that I should have the surgery as soon as possible. They said the risk of waiting for the surgery far outweighed the risk of being too large to be operated on. The Cleveland Clinic did say that there was a 7% increased chance of death during surgery due to my weight, but they, along with the other doctors, felt that my survivability depended on quick action to correct the blocked arteries. They all agreed that I had suffered a heart attack and needed to prevent another one, or worse.

When it was all said and done, I had reached a few conclusions. The first was that I could have the heart surgery safely done here in the Las Vegas area. The second is that there were some great surgeons here also. The third was that the hospital where I was to have my surgery was considered to be a very good hospital for cardiac surgery and the coronary care unit and intensive care unit to be top notch.

I picked a surgeon to do my surgery. His name was Dr. V.C. Smith. He had an outstanding reputation as a surgeon, and he ran what was considered by many the best surgical team and coronary care unit in the area. He was head of the cardiac surgery unit at St. Rose Dominican Hospital, Sienna Campus. He had just completed successful bypass surgery on the head basketball coach from the University of Nevada at Las Vegas.

When I first met him, he made me feel relaxed, and he understood my case. He had clearly examined all the films and charts that were forwarded for his review.

The hospital was relatively new to the area. St. Rose Dominican Hospital, Sienna Campus, was also known to have a good ICU (Intensive Care Unit) and coronary care unit. The hospital was very clean and well maintained. I have nothing but great things to say about the hospital and most of the services I received. The hospital was set up well so that my sister would be able to spend a great deal of time with me and be as comfortable as possible under the circumstances. The regular rooms were individual and allowed her to stay the night to keep an eye on me, as well as my medical caretakers. It was a very family-friendly hospital.

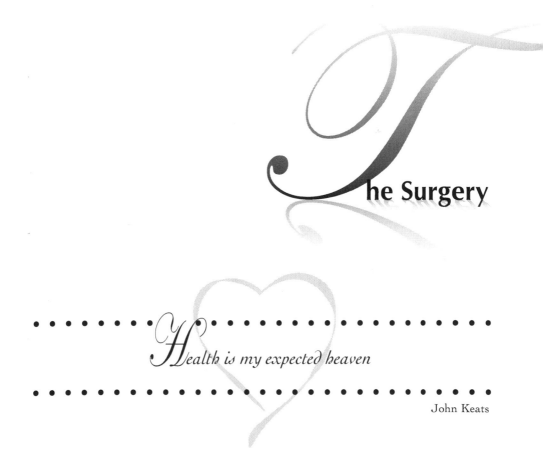

The Surgery

Health is my expected heaven

John Keats

August 23, 2007, was the big day. Leading up to that, I had a couple of very anxious weeks. Just knowing that you have to have such a serious medical procedure can be overwhelming to say the least. After I had interviewed and selected my surgeon, I remember the surgeon's office calling me two days later and telling me they had scheduled the surgery for the following week. I kind of freaked out. I thought it would be at least a couple of weeks. I could tell the person scheduling me knew that I was a little freaked. I told her there was no way on such short notice I could do that. She told me that she would have to check with the doctors and hospital schedule and see if it could be pushed back a week.

I had waited three and a half months, and now it was finally going to happen. I knew this was coming, but now it was the real deal. I was in no hurry, but when you need heart surgery, everything moves fast. I remembered going directly into my boss Jimmy's office with tears in my eyes and telling him they wanted to do surgery the following week. He told me to calm down and relax. He helped me put things in perspective as only he can do.

On a scale of 1 to 10, my anxiety level was a 20. As it turned out, the surgeon's office called back and was able and willing at my request to push the surgery back a week to August 23. That came as some relief, but I was still a little anxious. At that point someone told me that I needed something for my anxiety and should call my doctor. I was prescribed an anti-anxiety pill, and it seemed to help a lot. It took the edge off, if you will. I was able to sleep better and relax more. I couldn't take the medication during the day, however, because it made me tired.

A few days before the surgery, I remember not feeling well and feeling a little chest pressure. I thought it was in my head, but in hindsight I should have had it checked out. They probably would have admitted me to the hospital then. I tell everyone that if they feel any chest pressure, pain, or warning signs before their doctor's appointment or hospital visit to seek immediate medical attention. It is not something to play around with, and I would much rather be told that everything is OK than drop dead of a heart attack.

Recently, on a Monday night, I was out to dinner with a close friend who has diabetes and has been feeling some chest pressure with exertion while walking up stairs. He went to the doctor and was referred to his cardiologist that next Friday for what I assume was a stress test. I had told him that if he feels the heavy pressure before his scheduled appointment that he should go to the hospital. It turns out that the next day on Tuesday, he felt a lot of pressure and called his doctor. His doctor wisely told him to go to the emergency room. He went and after they performed an angiogram, he was told he had at least one artery 99% blocked. My point is "Do not mess around with warning signs!"

Another one of my friends called me on a Sunday morning to tell me his mother, who is 76 years old, just had five bypasses. It was emergency surgery. She had emphysema and thought all her chest pressure was a result of her bad lungs. It turns out that her heart was far worse than she thought. Thank goodness she got to the hospital in time.

There are several things you have done before being admitted to the hospital for surgery. In my case, I had to have chest x-rays, blood work, breathing tests, and an ultra-sound of my carotid arteries in the neck. The breathing tests were interesting because they measure lung capacity and the ability to suck in and blow out air. This is important because they need you to breathe while recovering from surgery. Expanding your lungs is a good way to keep pneumonia away and help speed up the recovery process. The first thing the nurse asked me was if I was a smoker. A smoker's recovery time and potential complications from surgery rise dramatically after surgery. Thank goodness I didn't smoke. I have dedicated a chapter on the health benefits of smoking in this book, so you will have to read on.

Everything was set. I was to be at the hospital at 5:00 a.m. My sister was going to be with me. I had prepared a list of people I wanted her to call following my surgery to let them know I was OK. One of my best friends, Glen, was at the hospital too to make sure I was OK. He later told me that he went into the ICU to see me after surgery and that when he saw me pee through my catheter into the bag, he told the doctors I would be fine. It was nice knowing he was looking out for me.

There are so many little booklets that the surgeon's office and hospital give you to read about open-heart surgery. From what to expect before, during, and after surgery, these booklets even talk about the impact on any caregiver or family that is around. There is a great deal of information on the surgical procedure itself. These booklets were very good to read and helped me through the process of knowing what to expect. Recovery is a main focus in these booklets also. The information is for the patient as well as any family member or caregiver. I can't stress enough that the more informed a patient is before entering the hospital, the better recovery will be.

When I got to the hospital, I went to admitting. I should note that the morning of the surgery I weighed 356 pounds. They put a wristband on me for identification. We were then directed to the waiting area to wait for the surgical prep team to call. It was about five in the morning, and we were sitting in the waiting area. There was a family that we could hear but not see that was sitting around the corner being consoled by social workers at the hospital. I could hear loud crying and uncontrollable sobbing. They had a loved one that was in an accident or something that was in critical condition in the ICU. Every ten minutes or so, a couple of the family members would walk past me, to and from the ICU, crying and holding on to one another. I could only conclude that they were told that this person may not make it, and they had to go give their prayers. I felt they were told to say their goodbyes to someone they loved. It was very difficult to witness this scene, but it was part of my day. It put many things into perspective. I don't know how things turned out with that family, but I knew it was in someone else's hands.

About an hour and a half went by, and I was called into the prep area. I had a Tau cross that my aunt Anneta had made and given to my mother. I had taken it when my mother had passed away and wore it every day. They made me take it off, and I made sure that Candy kept it near me all the time while I was in the hospital. I needed to know my mom was close.

The surgical prep team had two ladies that prepped patients for surgery. When you go into the room, they have you strip and put on a gown. Then they shaved my chest hairs, all three of them, and my legs. The legs are shaved because they use a vein from the leg as a graft for the artery bypasses. They can also use a vein from the chest. There are other procedures but this is how they did mine.

Once shaved, I was sent to the sterile shower area to shower with special soap. The soap sterilizes the body and primarily the surgical entry points. After the shower, I went back and lay down and waited for the nurse. My sister was in the room at this time waiting with me. I was trying to relax and was really at peace. I was thinking this could be someone else I know. Better me in this situation since I knew I could handle it. A nurse from the surgical team came in, and I remember her asking a few questions, then starting an IV.

The nurse told me that immediately following surgery I would have a breathing tube down my throat when I woke up. She said it would be removed as soon as I was alert and awake and breathing on my own after surgery. It was soon after that that my sister kissed me goodbye, squeezed my hand, and told me everything would be ok. I knew she was there representing all of my family. They took me to the operating room. They wheeled me not far from where I was, and all I could see was the ceiling. I did see a few heads when we got into the room and the anesthesiologist introduced himself.

Then It was Lights Out!

I suppose the surgery took a few hours, and I do remember waking up and having the tube pulled out of my throat. Everything else was sketchy for a while. I was in the ICU for a couple of days. I told my sister to limit visits from friends to just a couple of minutes and under no circumstances was there to be a cell phone near the room. The last thing

I wanted was to hear a stupid cell phone go off while I was recovering. Candy was with me most of the time at my bedside, but they did make her leave at night while I was in the ICU. I was kind of glad for that because she must have been exhausted, and I am sure she needed a break.

The first night I remember a great nurse who was next to my bed every minute. I think that the first night after heart surgery is the most critical, so they assign a one-on- one nurse. The nurse for my first night in ICU was Tori. She was no more than three feet from me the whole night. She was outstanding, and I felt lucky to have her by my side. She was very comforting with her words and professional care. I think nurses get the shaft most of the time and almost never get the recognition they deserve. A good nurse works so hard, and they have to do things so many of us would dread to do. I told all my nurses how much I appreciated them and always thanked them for their care.

I have always had a bad back and underwent back surgery to repair a disk some 10 years prior. I found it very difficult to lie in the bed. I was so uncomfortable. My back was just killing me while I was in the bed. That's saying a lot because of the pain medications I was on. During my stay in the hospital, I lay in a recliner chair most of the time. They were able to accommodate this need even in my regular room at the hospital.

I remember that I had no feeling in my right hand after the surgery. My hand felt numb. It took three days for the feeling to start to come back. It was explained to me that the reason for this loss of feeling was because my hand was most likely pinned underneath my body during the operation. I was told that in open-heart surgery, you are positioned like a butter-flied chicken with its wings pinned back.

When Dr. Smith, the surgeon, visited me in the room the next day after surgery, he said the surgery went well and that the grafts took well and looked strong. He did say he looked at my heart and turned it over and did not see any visible damage to the front or back of the heart. This news was a relief because until they actually see the heart, it's sometimes hard to tell the extent of any permanent damage. Remember that if the heart muscle is damaged during a heart attack, it does not regenerate itself. The damage is done and only prevention of further damage is what needs to be addressed. I was very lucky that my prognosis was so good.

While in the ICU, I noticed it was hard to take a deep breath. This is primarily due to two drainage tubes that come out just below the bottom of the incision and a few inches above the belly button. The drainage tubes, as I understand it, go back and underneath the lungs and heart. The tubes are left there for a day or two and are then removed. Once they are removed, you are one step closer to leaving the ICU. I remember that the surgical doctor on call came in my room and had me lie on the bed. She basically told me to exhale at the count of three and she would remove the tubes. I remember the relief of being able to take a deep breath after she pulled the tubes out. I had my eyes shut the whole time.

It was time for me to be transferred to a regular room. I was in the hospital from Thursday morning until Wednesday afternoon the following week. I had a lot of visitors. My oxygen level was low, so the nurses advised me that I needed to rest more. They said I needed to limit the duration and number of my visits and not talk so much. That has always proven difficult for me. I love to talk and entertain. I always have a lot to say. I knew that my recovery and getting out of the hospital were priorities, so I tried to listen to the nurses.

The support I had from family and friends was fantastic, and at times overwhelming. There are three things you don't want to do after open-heart surgery: sneeze, laugh, or cough. They are the most painful things you can experience. Believe you me, I can't describe the pain. I am allergic to certain perfumes and some floral scents. The last thing I wanted to do was sneeze. I had all the flowers that were sent to my room from friends given to the nurse's station or to another patient who had none on the floor.

The hospital staff gave me my heart pillow. This was a small but firm red heart-shaped pillow that you brace against your sternum when you move or feel as if you will sneeze or cough. You hold it tightly and close to your sternum when you move in certain directions. It was my best friend when I got in and out of bed. It becomes part of you. I was inseparable from my heart pillow for about six weeks after my surgery. My pillow was never more than arm's length away from me at any given moment. It is also something you keep next to your chest when you are in a car for added protection in case of an accident. Remember: my sternum was just sawed in half. I would hold it tightly to my sternum underneath the shoulder seat belt. I was lucky that I only sneezed infrequently in the few weeks after surgery. My mom always told me to hold my upper lip just below my nose between my thumb and forefinger for a moment to stop a sneeze. I don't know why, but Mother always had tricks that worked.

About three weeks out of surgery, I was watching a comedy movie at home with Candy while I was sitting in my recliner. A funny moment occurred, and I lost it. I started laughing so hard I began to cry from the pain. She started to laugh too. I held that pillow so tight against my chest, but it hurt like crap. It was just one of those moments. She turned the movie off. After I regained my composure, we restarted the movie. When the scene came up that broke me up before, it was just as funny as the first time. I began laughing and crying again. It would have been a favorite funny You Tube moment. She stopped the movie again. I think we finished it a week or two later.

I remember being in the room and even in ICU, and it seemed like they were taking x-rays and blood all the time. Physical therapy in the hospital is critical to recovery. The next day after surgery while in ICU, they get you out of bed, or in my case out of my recliner, and you start to walk. It hurts, but you must move after surgery. The first time I walked, I felt like I had just run a marathon. I think I walked with a walker and the therapist about seven feet to the door and then back to the chair. It seemed that it took all my energy just to do that. They came two times a day to get me to walk. Each time I tried to push myself more. I remember my physical therapist had to keep telling me to keep my head up while I was walking. You get disoriented and dizzy when you look down and not straight ahead. She had to tell me to breathe also. It's the little things that seem so large in recovery.

When I was in my room, I just wanted to walk a little farther each time. As a cardiac patient at the hospital, you receive a portable heart monitor for the nurse's station to monitor your vitals while you are walking with the therapist. I think the better shape you are in before you have surgery, the easier recovery will be. This probably goes for any surgery. One of the booklets I read before the surgery showed a drawing of how to get out of a bed and chair to stand up. I remember for a week before surgery sitting down and standing up over and over on the side of my bed to strengthen my legs and posture. I really believe this made a difference when I was at the hospital.

It was finally time to go home. I was so big I knew I had to work harder than someone who was in better physical shape...

...But I knew I could do it!

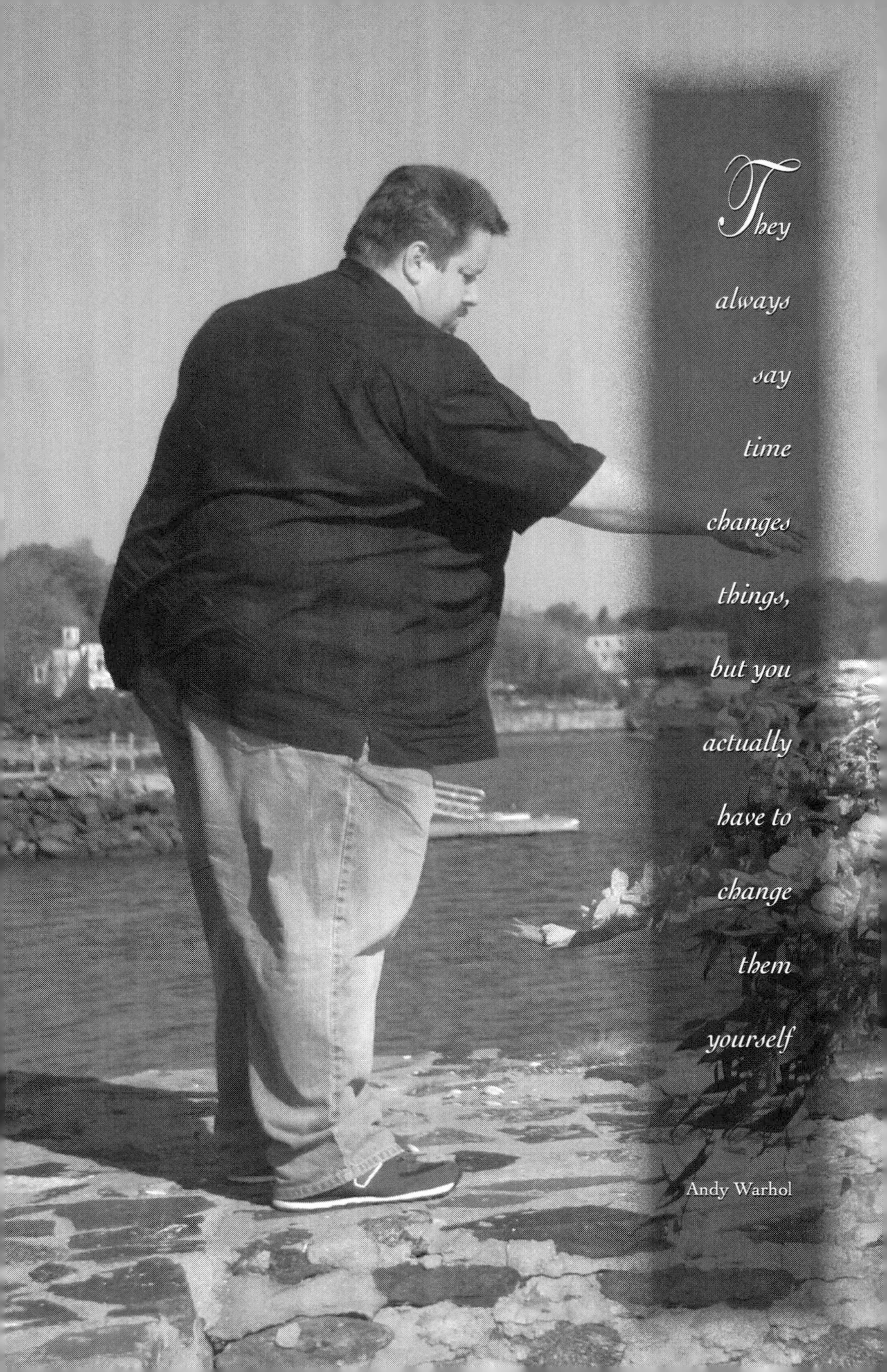

They

always

say

time

changes

things,

but you

actually

have to

change

them

yourself

Andy Warhol

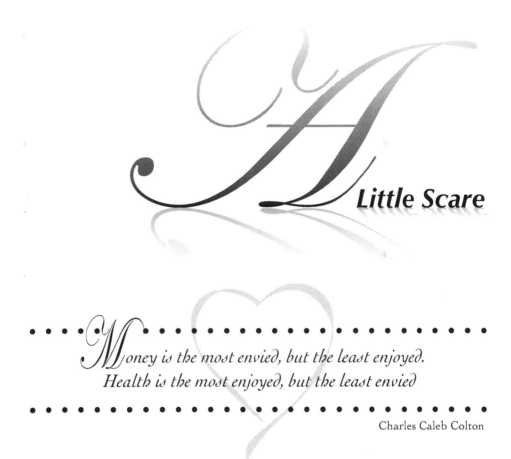

A Little Scare

Money is the most envied, but the least enjoyed.
Health is the most enjoyed, but the least envied

Charles Caleb Colton

I got home from the hospital on a Wednesday, and things seemed as if they were going according to plan. My friend Kem came to visit me on the Sunday after I was home. He stayed for a couple of hours and then left around 6 p.m. We had a nice visit, and I needed the company and my sister had a few errands to run.

I had to wear compression stockings at home for a while to prevent blood clots. They were so tight, and I remember my sister struggling each time to get them on me. Somehow she gathered the strength and put them on each time. It was about 8 p.m. that night and I was going to take a shower before trying to go to bed. Kem had just left a couple of hours earlier. Candy was getting ready to take the stockings off, and I just didn't feel right. I had some abnormal pain in my upper chest, and I could feel my heart beat each time. It was a very strange and unnatural feeling. I was getting concerned. I kept how I was feeling to myself for about 20 minutes or so thinking the pain would go away.

As Candy was about to take the stockings off I told her not to. I described the feelings I was having to her. I told her I thought we should call the doctor. She knew I was serious because a few days before the surgery, I was having some pains and she wanted to call the doctor and I told her no. She called the cardiologist's office, and because it was a Sunday night, she left a message with the answering service. A couple minutes later, before we could hear back from the doctor, I told her that I thought we should go to the hospital. I was a little scared and the feeling was not going away.

She calmly collected a few things and I managed to get in the car. Candy kept very calm throughout this event, and I am sure it helped me stay somewhat relaxed. We drove to the hospital, which is about 15 minutes from the house, and I got out of the car at the emergency entrance. I walked in and Candy parked the car. I had my heart pillow in tow. They sat me down in a wheelchair and I remember the emergency room being packed. I explained that I had just had surgery and what I was feeling. A nurse came out pretty quickly, and the staff started to assess my situation. The nurses took blood and they did an EKG right away.

I was feeling a little anxious at this time. I was put on a bed and taken to the emergency room to a stall. They started to monitor me and gave me a few shots of something. The emergency room nurse kept putting warm blankets on me. I remember being so cold. I remember after seeing the ER doctor they gave me a couple more shots in the stomach area. Later I was to find out that this was blood thinner. It was all preventative. The doctor wanted to do a test that involved a scan but he told me I was too large for this particular machine. He had to do another test, but it would not be as quick to diagnose the problem. Candy sat next to me the whole time.

The doctor told me that my symptoms indicated a pulmonary embolism, a blood clot in the pulmonary artery near the heart. The blood thinner was given to prevent the clot from dislodging or getting bigger. He was waiting for a team to come in to do a test on me that would help him determine if this indeed was what was happening. The doctor left the stall.

There was a lady in the next stall screaming in pain from an injury or illness. I tried my best to zone everything out that was happening around me. I was lying there staring at the ceiling, and I started to cry. I remember Candy wiping tears out of my eyes and reassuring me everything would be ok. It was the only time I can honestly say that I was scared and afraid. I knew that a blood clot, if that's what it was, is dangerous. I kept thinking to myself, *Could this be it? Is this how I was going to check out?* I was thinking that I had just undergone major heart surgery and came out OK. I was so afraid that they were going to have to cut my chest open again. I remember telling Candy that at least all my affairs were in order should something happen.

The nurse came back shortly, although it seemed like days, and they wheeled me to another room. There was a team of three people, and they put me in what I would describe as a scanner. It reminded me of an MRI machine. I was told not to move and they would get different scans of my chest. The test was completed, and I was returned to the ER. The results revealed that I did not have an embolism, thank the Lord.

I think I took my first breath in four hours.

They were not sure what it was that was causing my pain, but they ruled out the worst case scenario. They were going to admit me to the hospital for observation, and I was to see a cardiologist the next day. It was about 3:00 a.m., and I got into the regular room. I remember it was next to the pediatric ICU.

The nurse for my room that night was great. I thought that she would never understand a heart patient, but as it turned out, she explained to me she had had a heart attack a year earlier and was doing fine. She understood my situation, and I felt so much better. I felt a lot better the next day, and the symptoms had gone away. The cardiologist came to see me the next day and said that the pain and discomfort that I was feeling was post surgical and that some patients experience these symptoms. He could not see any other problems with me. I felt like an ass, but he told me clearly that I did the right thing by getting to the hospital right away. He told me that it could have been very serious and that the decision to go to the emergency room was a good one. I was discharged and went home a couple of hours later.

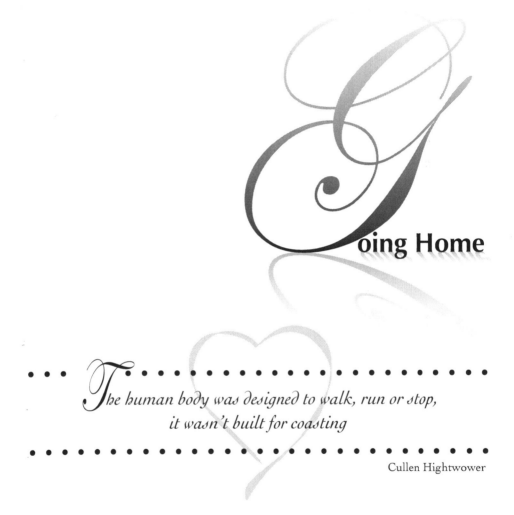

Going Home

The human body was designed to walk, run or stop, it wasn't built for coasting

Cullen Hightwower

I have a two-story home with a very big staircase. I thought it would be easier to stay downstairs for recovery. I was able to get a hospital bed delivered under my insurance. There is a large shower downstairs also. My recliner is also downstairs. I had a good setup, given the circumstances.

At home, as in the hospital, you have to move around. Walking seems to speed all post surgical recovery. My sister made me get up at least twice a day and walk around the house. I have a large statue of a saxophone guy in the living room and a pinball machine in the family room next to my bed. I would take 5 quarters and put them on the pinball machine. I took one quarter at a time and walked it to the saxophone guy and put it on the saxophone bell. It was probably about 25 steps. I then walked back to the pinball machine and got another quarter and repeated this until all the quarters had been moved. I eventually worked my way up to 10 quarters going back and forth.

After a week or so, I started to walk outside. I used a walker just for mental support and would go a little farther each day. My walker had a sitting area on it in case I got tired, and my heart pillow was always with me. I was so afraid of sneezing with the pollen in the air. The good thing is that I got my sister to walk with me. I knew this did her good too. I tried to maintain a very balanced and healthy selection of food during my recovery, and Candy would make her homemade chicken soup each week: it was probably my best medicine.

I made a little progress each day. You kind of go crazy after a while sitting at home all day. I just wanted to get back to work. My friend Jim came over a couple of days to sit with me while my sister took a break and went to the store. Jim would walk with me up the stairs. I remember him telling me I had to put one foot in front of the other. My friend Jim had multiple stents put in his heart, so he was the closest friend I had who could even relate to what I was going through. My friends were so generous with their time. I knew how much my sister needed a break also.

There were a couple nights I remember when I woke up in the middle of the night freezing. I must have gotten the chills and my teeth were chattering. Candy got up and was heating sheets and extra blankets in the dryer to put over me to keep me warm. Open-heart surgery is trauma if you think of it. Your body is put through so much.

The days seemed to go by OK, but sometimes the pain was awful. There is a lot of healing with open-heart surgery, and your body is recovering minute by minute. There were good hours and crappy hours, good days and bad days. I did learn that you should control pain before it gets very bad. Post surgery, they say that when pain is coming on to take your medicine so it doesn't get out of hand. I was as stubborn as the next guy when it comes to being macho and learned by trial and error, mostly by error, that it pays to control the pain.

I was at home for exactly four weeks after surgery before going back to work. I went back for a few hours a day. I probably pushed it a little because I remember being so tired and run down when I got home. In hindsight I wish I had taken six weeks off before going back. It is recommended that you don't drive for at least six weeks after open-heart surgery. I didn't have to drive for about eight weeks because I had my sister and a co-worker or two helping me. You just can't react if you need to avoid an accident, and the steering wheel is too close to your sternum in case of a sudden stop. It was still challenging for a while to get in and out of a car. It hurt badly to move when you got in and out of a car. My heart pillow was always with me and tight against my body when I was getting in and out of a car. I was lucky I had a desk job. I imagine so many people have such a hard time going back to work especially if they have to lift things or do manual labor. I was real lucky.

I continued to progress a little each day with normal setbacks. I was able to eventually move into my bed upstairs. One of the things that was so difficult was sleeping on my back because I have always slept on my side or stomach. It was very uncomfortable, and I was very restless to say the least trying to sleep on my back. Because I was so large, there was always extra pressure on my chest when I attempted to turn on my side. The pain at times was excruciating. However, about 14 weeks after surgery, I was able to turn on my side and sleep more comfortably.

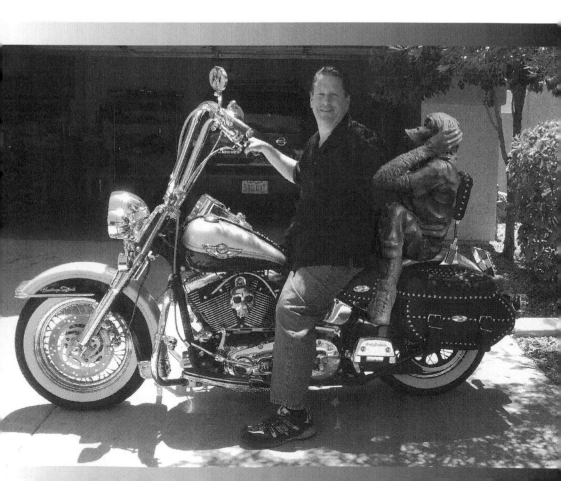

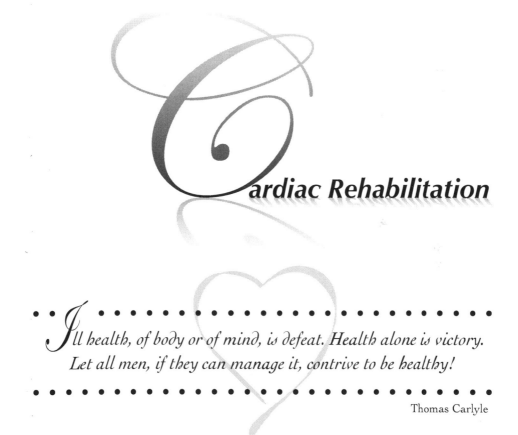

Cardiac Rehabilitation

*Ill health, of body or of mind, is defeat. Health alone is victory.
Let all men, if they can manage it, contrive to be healthy!*

Thomas Carlyle

Cardiac rehabilitation can start as early as six weeks from open-heart surgery. The six weeks are needed to allow time for the sternum to heal. My hospital offered cardiac rehabilitation for patients that had heart or stroke issues. These issues included, but were not limited to, open heart surgery, stents, strokes, and so on. I found the program incredibly valuable and couldn't figure out why anyone would not take advantage of it. I understand that most insurance companies cover such treatment for a period of time. If insurance didn't pay for it, it would be practically impossible to attend because of the cost. Excluding insurance issues, I would highly recommend a cardiac rehabilitation program to anyone who could benefit from it.

After talking with other patients and nurses, I was distraught to find out that not all doctors were gung ho about their patients attending. I still can't figure this one out. If they only knew how much it helped me. These are really the classes where the old cliché comes into play that you only get out of something what you put into it. I looked forward to the classes because I just knew they were going to help me.

The program started me on an exercise program that I could continue after the class ended. In my case, I was in the class for about twelve weeks. In the class, a monitor measures your heart rate and rhythm; your blood pressure is checked throughout the exercises. Two exercise physiologists attended each session along with registered nurses to make sure your technique was good and for the obvious medical care if needed.

Stretching is a major part of the program. They showed me how important it was to stretch and warm up BEFORE and AFTER my workout. I still do the same stretches today. The nurses were also available for nutrition information. The exercise part of the program involved four fitness exercises. The fitness exercises were treadmill, exercise bike, ergometer, and weight training. The ergometer is the machine that is like a bicycle but you pedal it with your hands. It helps with regaining mobility in your arms and chest and develops upper body strength.

I remember going to the class for the first time. I was still in a lot of discomfort at times and was not sleeping well. I felt intimidated because some of the people were moving like athletes. There was a guy that was running on the treadmill. I was thinking I could never do that. I was still sleeping on my back because it hurt too much to sleep on my side. When you get to a class, you have to keep in mind that everyone is on a different level. Some of the people are ready to graduate, and others have just started, like me. I had to take the program one day at a time. I later found out that the guy who was running like a champ on the treadmill was recovering from a stroke. Before the stroke he was running six miles a day. Because you are so well monitored during your rehabilitation, your individual progress is easy to see. Progress reports are completed by the nurse after each session and sent to your doctors weekly. The cardiac rehabilitation program was fantastic. I am so happy and proud I attended and completed the course.

The following is a letter I sent to the hospital administrators to show my appreciation for my cardiac rehabilitation team and the invaluable rehabilitation experience I had.

January 13, 2008

Mr. Rod Davis, President and Chief Executive Officer
Ms. Teressa Conley, Chief Operating Officer
Dr. V.C. Smith, MD., F.A.C.S.
St. Rose Dominican Hospital - Siena Campus
3001 St. Rose Parkway, Henderson, NV 89052

Dear Mr. Davis, Ms Conley, and Dr. Smith,

I want to express my appreciation and gratitude for attending and graduating from the St. Rose Dominican Hospital Cardiopulmonary Rehabilitation program on North Green Valley Parkway. I had a heart attack and was a Cardiac Bypass Patient of Dr. V.C. Smith, MD. and Cardiologist Dr. Leo Spaccavento, MD.

This program was outstanding. It saw me through the difficult first stage of getting me back on my feet to feeling like a leader in the class because of my cardio workout accomplishments.

It is very important that the Directors of St. Rose recognize the outstanding work and dedication of the entire staff of the Rehab team.

The main team during my rehab included registered nurses Jackie and Kathy and exercise physiologists Emily and Keri. Each was great and professional while making the classes fun to attend. They sure know their business.

I must give special thanks and recognition to Jackie, the lead R.N., who always kept things moving and motivating in the classes. During a very difficult time for me when my father passed away, she showed incredible compassion and caring while keeping me focused. She is an asset to any hospital or health care facility when so much is at stake. You are lucky to have her.

This group of individuals helped me start my " New Life." I don't intend on letting them or myself down. I will continue the path they have set me on.

Thank you for being there for me.

With great respect and admiration,
Keith A. Ahrens
cc: Dr. Leo Spaccavento

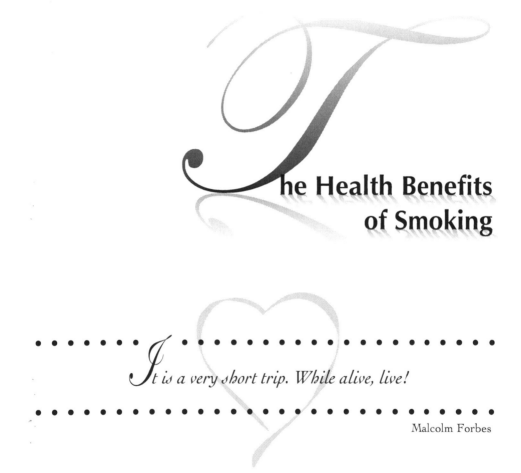

The Health Benefits of Smoking

It is a very short trip. While alive, live!

Malcolm Forbes

There are none.

Smoking will make you sick.

Smoking will kill you one cigarette at a time.

It will seriously harm those around you.

Quit smoking now and you will live longer and be healthier.

Smoking is a major risk factor in heart disease.

The reason for this chapter is that I hate smoking. I am seriously allergic to cigarette smoke and have been since I was a child. I also have read too many bad things about the correlation of smoking and heart disease and cancer. For some reason, I am super sensitive to second-hand smoke, even to the extent that if someone just smoked and it is on their breath, it will disturb me. I have had to explain for years when people entered my office and had just smoked that they would need to use a breath mint or gum before I could continue speaking with them. I wasn't trying to be rude, although that's how many perceived it. I was just trying not to get sick. I hate being in the presence of cigarette smoke. The second-hand smoke gives me an immediate headache, and I always feel sick when I am around smoke. I get a sick feeling even when I am around ashtrays, indoors or outdoors.

End of Chapter.

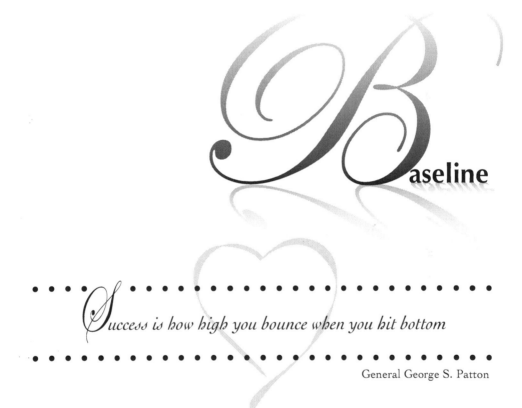

Baseline

We have all seen the disclaimers on the exercise equipment we use or on the television infomercials. You know, the one that says, "Consult a physician before beginning any exercise program." We even see the same disclaimer on so many diet programs. It is on some of the medicines we take. I am here to tell you it is there for a reason. After what I went through, I am a big proponent of getting your doctor's OK to start any exercise program. You have to have a checkup. You need to know that you are medically OK to proceed and work out. Besides that, you are doing it for a reason. At the very least you will be able to better track your overall progress. Results are the key to keeping on track and keeping you motivated.

I use the word *baseline* to describe where you are now as far as the vital medical statistics you want to track. Before you start any successful weight loss, diet, physical fitness, or exercise program, the key is knowing what your baseline is or what your beginning vital medical statistics are, such as cholesterol, triglycerides, blood pressure, pulse rate, or any other potential medical issues. Your success will be measured by your progress both physically and medically. Don't underestimate the positive, motivating results of regular blood work and checkups that have improved over time. Improvement and being able to track your success are very motivating. I find that keeping the good stuff good and improving on the stuff you are trying to change are very motivating. For me, it was my good or HDL cholesterol, which was very low and a major factor in my heart disease. I watched that number go from dangerously low to being in the normal range.

I love

to see the

numbers go up!

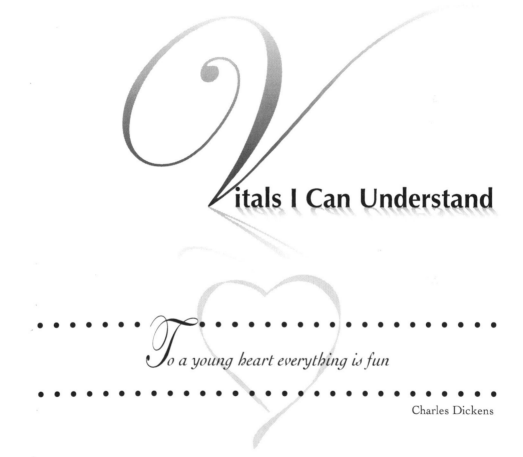

Vitals I Can Understand

To a young heart everything is fun

Charles Dickens

It is important to know where you stand and what targets you and your doctor want to achieve. By being diligent and working "your" plan, you will see results. Keep something in mind. It took you years to get where you are, so don't expect results overnight, but I believe you will be amazed at your progress if you keep track every few months. I was able to see my primary physician every three months and my cardiologist every six months. I have been able to monitor my weight loss and blood levels with these visits. There were some key medical numbers that I kept a very close eye on and will keep track of the rest of my life. You may have others that are not on my list that you need to monitor. I do not have diabetes and only get screened once a year at my annual physical. You may need to be screened more often.

The things that I monitor on a regular basis are:

Cholesterol – 3 elements

    Total cholesterol

    Good - HDL

    Bad - LDL

Triglycerides

Weight

Pulse rate

Blood pressure

At the end of the book, I am going to offer some informational charts and a few brief explanations of the items I monitor for myself. Remember that these items are to be used only as a general guide. **Ask your doctor what ranges you should be in. Only take medical advice from your doctor**. Keep in mind that you are part of your own medical team. Also, do your own research. I found that internet searches provided me with a wealth of information on almost any subject.

Eating Right:
My 95% – 5% Rule

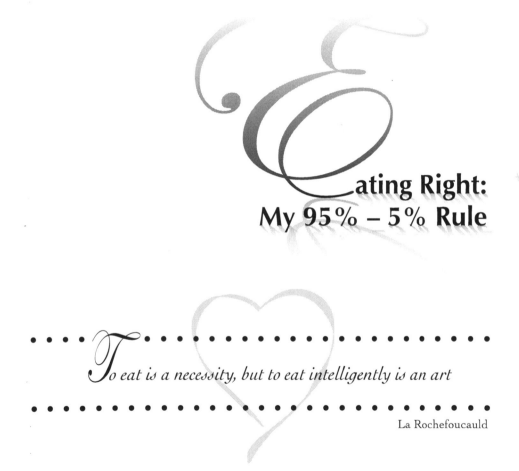

To eat is a necessity, but to eat intelligently is an art

La Rochefoucauld

"Nothing tastes as good as being thin feels."

I don't know who wrote it, but I remember someone saying it when I was on another yo-yo diet twenty-some years ago. But it sure holds true to this day.

Splurging and rewarding yourself occasionally are not the death of any weight loss plan. It is just the opposite in my opinion. Here's why: I had a craving for popcorn while I was in cardiac rehabilitation. I don't know why, but I wanted popcorn in the worst way. I was eating very healthy and didn't want to go off my plan. Emily, one of my exercise coaches, told me that the best thing to do was to go get myself some popcorn and eat some. Her feeling was that if I denied myself the popcorn that I wanted so badly, I would binge on something else in the fridge or pantry that I most likely didn't care about. She was probably right, and I did eat my popcorn that night. I try to satisfy my cravings when they occur, but I do it in moderation. I can still love the foods that I have always loved. But I had to put it in perspective for myself and make some changes.

I have adapted the following in my healthy eating plan: Instead of eating 95% crap and 5% good, I have been eating 95% good and 5% crap.

Let's face it; many of us eat so much garbage and try to justify it with a piece of fruit or a salad. Sorry, but that just doesn't cut it.

What I really hate is the salads offered at the fast food places with their terrible selection of complementary dressings. Go to a search engine on your computer and type in "fast food nutrition." It will make you rethink your order when you read the calorie or fat gram content of any of the fast foods we eat so much. I admit, I love them too, but it all boils down to the choices we make. I still can't figure out why these companies don't have simple balsamic or extremely low-calorie, low-fat dressings that taste good. When I was at work all the time, it was just too easy not to eat right. At work, we always seemed to be in a hurry and made so many bad choices. The convenience of fast food makes poor choices of food easy. I have found that some of the submarine sandwich shops post their nutritional information for their products. Some of the selections are actually pretty good. I have found myself using mustard instead of mayonnaise.

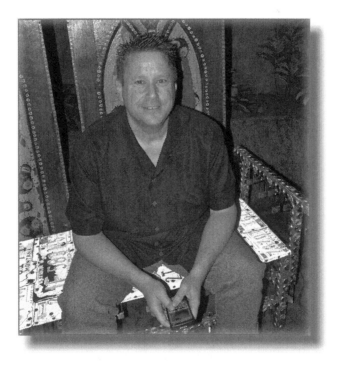

I am not a nutritionist or dietician, so I can only speak for myself as to what has worked for me. I think that the simpler it is, the better the results. There are so many heart-healthy and low-fat diet books out there. Go to the book store and pick up one or two cookbooks, or you can find and print hundreds of heart-healthy recipes online. They all have the same underlying principles, and that is low fat, low sodium, low calorie and high protein. Pretty simple isn't it? We just need to know what the ingredients are and modify them to our daily food choices. It isn't hard to understand that fruits and vegetables are good for you. Non-processed foods are better than processed foods. Skinless chicken is a wiser choice than beef. Water is good.

Lets get back to my 95% – 5% rule.

Think of it this way. Imagine you had a birthday every day or that it was Christmas every day. Imagine if you had to eat your favorite food every day. Pretty soon, it would be no big deal, and you would probably get tired of these days, and your favorite food would turn into your least desirable food.

Now let me relate that to food in general. If you eat healthy 95% of the time and you only splurge 5% of the time, the reward of the foods you eat will be greatly enhanced. I personally look forward to having cheese on some Sundays. I love artisan cheeses. I also have developed a taste for very dark chocolates. These foods are part of my 5% rule. I always try to eat in moderation, and I feel quite satisfied after I do. I feel so rewarded, and it doesn't feel as if I'm cheating as much as I am savoring something I love, and it is part of my reward for a good week of exercise and eating right.

I love grilled vegetables. I have found that eggplant, scallions, potatoes, bell peppers, pineapple, and—my favorite—asparagus, and just about anything you put on the grill tastes great. I use a little extra virgin olive oil and a little salt and pepper on most of my grilled veggies. I live in the desert of Nevada. I have found it hard to find good fresh vegetables. Don't take for granted a great fresh vegetable when you can get it. My sister Beth sent me a care package from her garden this summer, with tomatoes, bell peppers, squash, and some fresh, homemade salsa. The flavor and taste of fresh garden-grown and ripened veggies were just awesome. When I was eating the tomatoes, I felt as if I was eating a rib eye steak, they tasted so good.

I have turned into a chicken fanatic. I buy boneless skinless chicken breasts when they go on sale. I stock up so that I always have chicken in the house. I cook chicken so many ways it seems like I never eat it the same way. I experiment all the time. Grilled chicken and veggies are my favorite.

I have traveled to China twice since my heart surgery. The Chinese love spices. They know how to use them and use a large variety of peppers in their dishes. I was never a spicy food eater, but I have found my tastes have changed as I have lost weight. I seem to go through flavor phases. I really enjoy and like spicy foods now and then. I love to experiment with fresh and dried peppers in my cooking. Someone even told me that spices are good for the metabolism.

I have had cravings for beef, but have substituted ground buffalo to make an occasional burger. It tastes great, and if you look up the nutritional information on it, you will be amazed at the low-calorie, high-protein, and low-fat content of the meat. If you can find it, fresh ground buffalo meat is fantastic. You can find it frozen in a lot of stores, but fresh is best. I have been able to find ostrich a couple of times. It is great also and has outstanding nutritional value compared to beef. I found that not all meats have the same fat, protein, or calorie content as beef. I also discovered soy burgers. They are not as bad as they sound. Don't misunderstand me. I love a great steak on occasion, but it is in moderation and not often. I think that on the occasion that I do eat red meat, I appreciate a great steak more now than I ever did. I found that I do not miss my red meat as much as I thought I would. I used to eat a lot of red meat. The local steak houses used to love me. If you do eat beef, the filet has less fat, and if you do buy red meat, the cheaper grades like "select" or "choice" (as opposed to the more marbled and expensive prime cuts) are the ones we should be eating due to the amount of fat in the meat.

I try to eat as much fruit as I can. I eat a lot of bananas. I find the banana is filling and a great on-the-fly snack. I try to find fruit and eat what is in season. Great fruit in the desert of Nevada is hard to find, but I am always searching.

I eat a ton of cereal. I eat it in the morning with breakfast and often as dessert or a snack before bed. I can eat cereal anytime. It tastes great, and it is very filling. I only drink and use skim or fat free milk in my cereal. When I was eighteen, I was working out a lot and was concerned about protein and calories at the time. I developed a taste for skim milk as much as I know some people hate it. I find it hard now, if not impossible, to drink even 2% milk because of the fat content. Anything but skim milk to me feels like I am drinking fat. I feel fortunate that I took a liking to it for so many years.

Fish has become a part of my regular meals. I love tuna and salmon and all kinds of fish. I have found so many easy ways to prepare fish. Broiled and grilled are the best for me.

I drink a lot of water. I regularly drink about six, sixteen-ounce bottles of water throughout the day. I always drink after I workout and try to stay hydrated. Remember, I live in the desert, and it is normally very dry. I believe that water is a key element to any weight-loss program. I feel that keeping my body flushed and hydrated makes me feel better. You should ask your doctor how much water you should be drinking each day.

There is a snack bar on the market that has a high protein content of about 10 grams and is only 140 calories and is high in potassium. They also make the same bar that has 220 calories and 19 grams of protein. It comes in a few flavors that taste great. This bar has been a good midmorning or afternoon snack.

I have learned to read the labels of many food items for their nutritional content. There are so many resources online to learn about nutrition and nutritional content of so many foods. I know that when you work out the way I do, your body needs a lot of nutrition. Carbohydrates to give you energy and protein to rebuild muscles are just a few of the nutrients you need to keep going. Balance is the key. The bottom line is that you need to make choices in what you put into your mouth.

I am always asking myself

if I am making the right choices.

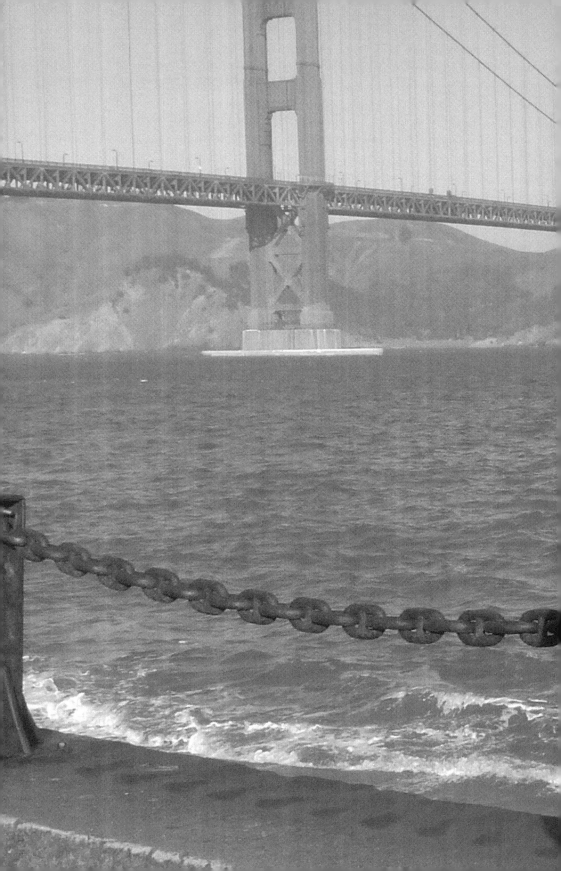

When I let go of what I am, I become what I might be

Lao Tzu

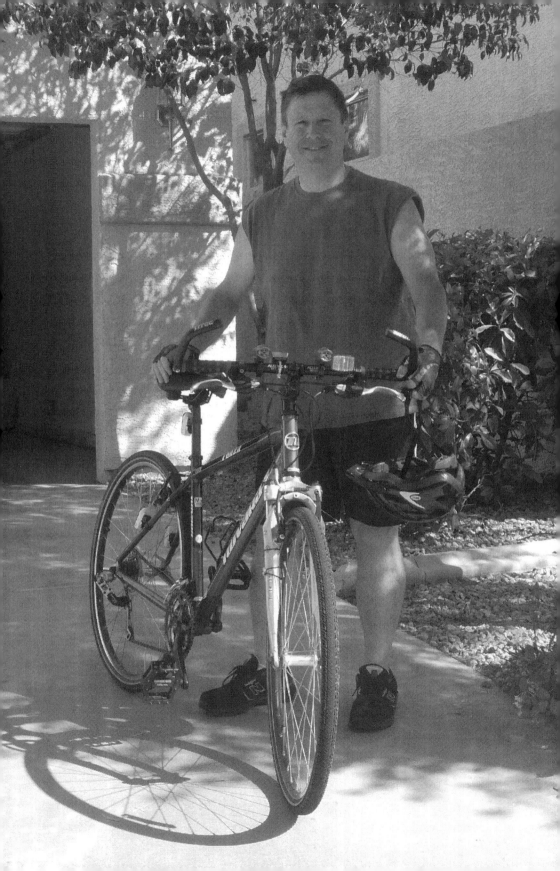

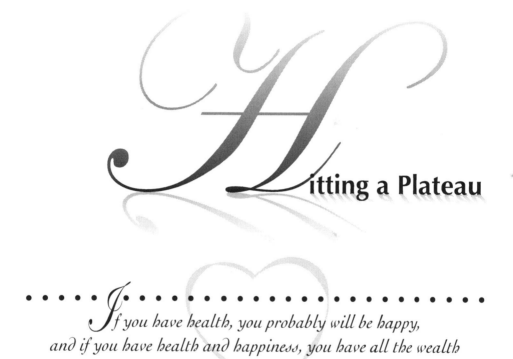

Hitting a Plateau

*If you have health, you probably will be happy,
and if you have health and happiness, you have all the wealth
you need, even if it is not all you want*

Elbert Hubbard

Hitting a plateau is a by-product and an inevitability of any weight-loss regimen. I hate hitting a plateau, but have had too many to count since watching what I was eating and exercising regularly and losing weight. It is very discouraging and in my opinion the biggest time and opportunity for the possibility of failure and going backwards. You feel like you have been eating right and exercising and your weight does not move down.

The reason for a plateau, they say, is because the body gets used to your exercise routine and or eating habits. I have found that when I plateau, I try to shake things up to jump-start my weight loss. I will attempt to exercise and eat differently. Your body has gotten used to your

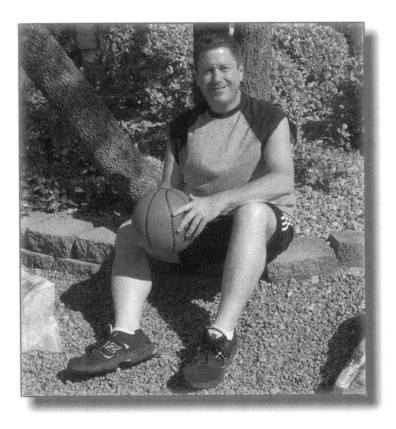

typical routine and is begging for something different. I will eat more or less food, and try to exercise on a different machine or maybe do a bicycle ride instead of walking on the treadmill. If I have been eating a lot of fruit, I may decide to eat more carbohydrates or move from carbo-hydrates to more protein. I may try this for three or four days, and I find that this often helps.

I have lost a lot of weight, and at first when you are so big, it seems to come off a lot faster. Now it seems it is harder to lose weight, and I find myself having to refocus often to stay on track. I must stay determined and realize that I am doing the right things to lose more weight and be more fit. Plateaus can last a few days or a few weeks or longer. I just stay smart and focused knowing I am doing the right things, and I should be back on track.

A lot of people ask me how often I weigh myself.

It's a good question.

I weigh myself once a week, at the same time each week. If I forget to weigh myself in my regular routine, I will wait until the follow-ing week to get back on the scale. On Sunday mornings, I wake up and before I eat or drink anything or work out I will go downstairs and step on the scale. I never get on the scale other than my regular time. I want to make sure I get a regular reading at the same time each week. I think it is important to weigh yourself on a regular basis to track your progress...

...*But I don't believe*

you should be obsessed with it!

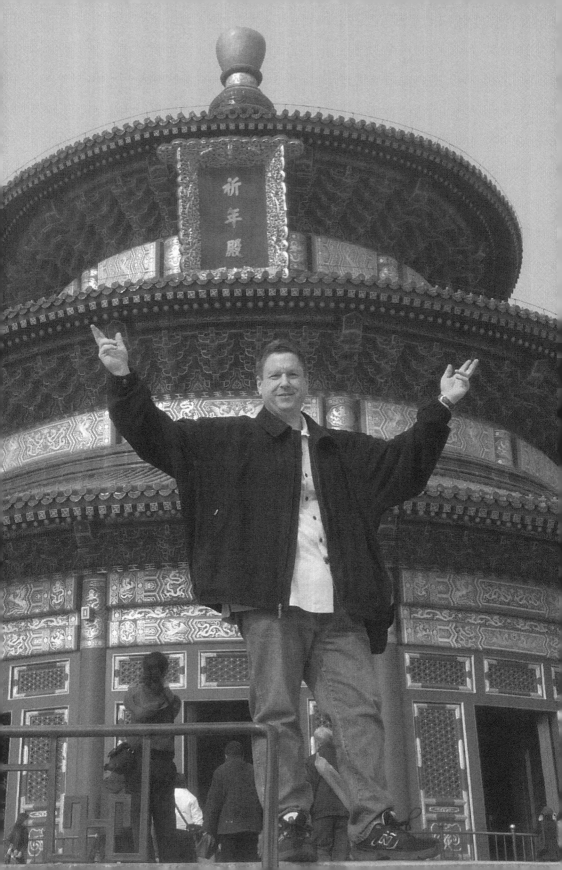

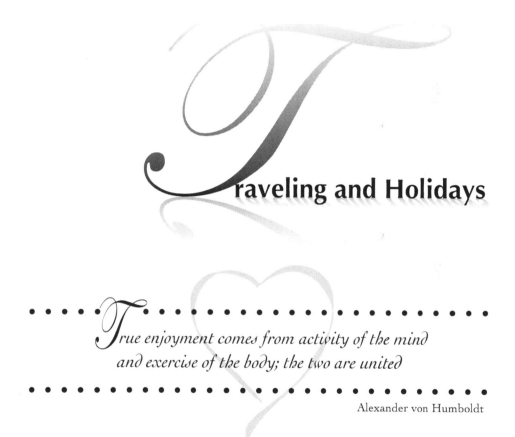

Traveling and Holidays

True enjoyment comes from activity of the mind and exercise of the body; the two are united

Alexander von Humboldt

Traveling and holidays to me fall right in the same category. When I travel, it seems to me that half the fun is eating and tasting the local cuisines. I love to eat when I travel. Eating what the locals eat is part of my vacation. The holidays bring back the foods we love. Old family recipes are always great and evoke so many memories of the past. But traveling and holidays can be trying times when you are trying to lose weight and make healthy decisions.

Like most people, I seem to overeat when I travel or head home for the holidays. I recently had a double whammy. I went to San Francisco the day after Thanksgiving for a break, and then I went home to Maryland for the Christmas holiday. Thirty days of guilt, it seemed. My brother Bruce had cooked the ultimate Christmas holiday dinner. He had everything on the table and then some. I thought I was going to gain a hundred pounds. I did gain a couple pounds by the time I got home,

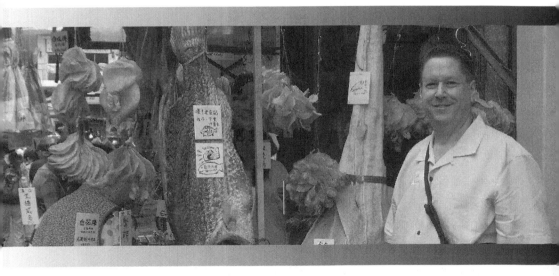

but knew I had to work it off. What's funny is that there are no free rides when losing weight. A pound is 3500 calories no matter how much or what we decide to eat.

I make sure that when I travel that there is a fitness gym or exercise machines at the hotel. I try to work out in the mornings no matter what. I say to myself that I will work out each day no matter what whenever I travel. It seems to ease the blow if and when I may indulge, if you will. I have recently changed my philosophy when I travel now that allows me to enjoy local foods. I simply try to concentrate on eating smaller portions of food. I try to put it in perspective, that even though I am away, I should still remember the principles of trying not to overeat and remember what I am trying to accomplish.

On my trip this February to Beijing, I was lucky to be upgraded and seated in business class. Now, in business class they serve three or sometimes four-course meals with all the snacks you can eat. I was very

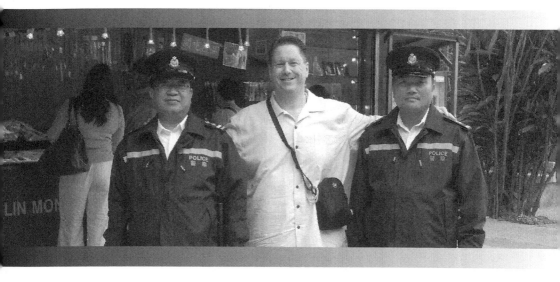

hungry because I had a very early connecting flight. If you haven't had airplane food in a while, let me tell you that the meals in first or business class are prepared and put together by some top-notch chefs. They are trying to make you feel like you are at a great restaurant 35,000 feet in the air.

It was now about 12:30 in the afternoon. I had gotten up at 3:30 a.m. and only had a protein bar at the airport. I had to make a connecting flight back in San Francisco. Before the flight took off, the flight attendant handed me a menu and asked me to select my entrée for my first meal. At first I picked braised short ribs with a demi-glace sauce. Now that sounded great and full of fat and calories. Before she left the cabin, I called her over and told her to switch my entrée to the chicken breast and assorted vegetables. A much wiser decision, I thought. Hell, I was on my way to Beijing to eat all the local foods. What did I need to fill up on the airline food for? In twelve and a half hours I would be in China. Two years ago, I was eating everything that was on the airplane and then some.

She came with the first course, which was a house tossed salad with tomatoes and red pepper. The appetizer was fresh smoked salmon, Genoa salami slices, raw broccoli and carrots, with a mayonnaise-based spicy creamy sauce on the side for dunking the veggies into. Two chunks of butter were in a side dish. The butter was for the roll she would soon offer me. When the salad was presented, she offered two dressing choices. One of the dressings was a Caesar salad dressing and the other was an oil-based balsamic vinaigrette dressing.

Now, I know how much fat the Caesar salad dressing has, and the heavy oil that I saw in the balsamic vinaigrette appeared just as bad. I told her I would pass on the dressing and eat my salad without it. When they offered me a roll for the butter, I politely said no to the roll because I knew that I would eat the butter. I ended up eating the salad with no dressing, which tasted just fine. I tapped the tomatoes into a dash of salt and pepper, and I ate the salmon and veggies that were on the plate. I left the salami and the spicy mayonnaise sauce on the plate, which looked great, I might add.

Not bad, I thought.

Now the entree came, and it was a boneless, skinless chicken breast roasted in a lemon and rosemary sauce with string beans, onions, and small red potato sections. *Good selection*, I thought again. For dessert she offered either tiramisu or two small cheese slices with purple wine grapes. I selected the cheese and wine grapes and only ate half the cheese and all the grapes. I can't tell you how much I wanted to eat the tiramisu.

Now why is this so significant? After my plates were cleared and I wiped my hands, I then realized I had done something that I had never done before on an airplane. I restrained from overeating, and I had just made some significantly healthier choices while in the air. I was actually so proud of myself that I teared up. It didn't matter if this was a new way of life, but I did realize that it was a special moment. It was a big moment for me, and that's all that mattered. And that moment can never be taken away from me. All of the little positive decisions that I have made have added up to one felt success after another.

When we travel or go home for the holidays, we just need to think about what we are eating and making sure we do everything to keep up with our physical-fitness routine.

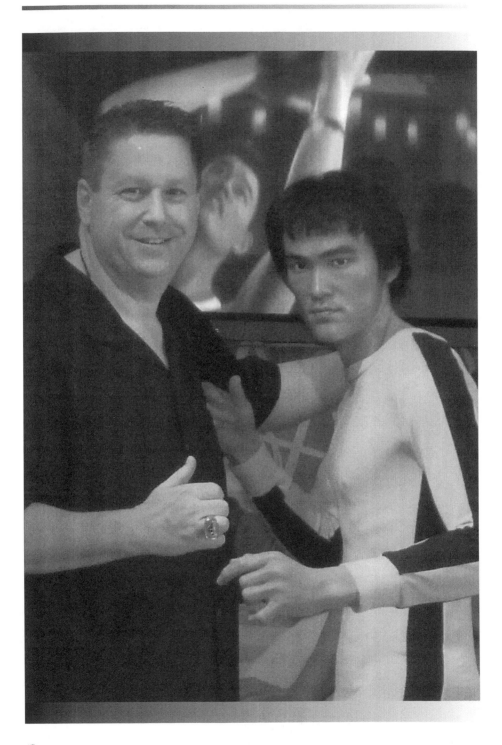

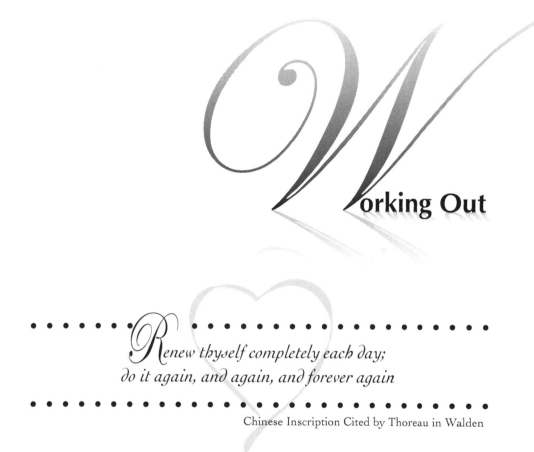

Working Out

I am not a fitness expert nor do I pretend to be. I do know that exercise is good and helps keep me healthy. The reason a gym has so many machines and exercise products is because what may work for you may not work for me.

Look at all of the television infomercials that tout one workout, machine, or exercise product over another. I believe that at some point, this particular product helped someone. It may or may not be for you. The health and fitness industry knows that the number-one reason someone quits using a piece of gym equipment at home or at the gym is because it is uncomfortable over time. Make sure that if you invest in any kind of gym equipment that you make every effort to try it out first. I was lucky with my stationary bicycle that the place I purchased it from had several on display, and I was able to try them out first. I actually did two twenty minute rides on the bike on separate days to make sure my bike was right for me.

When I began my exercise routine, I started walking for just five minutes at a time and became completely winded and struggled to get through the walk. I remember walking for ten minutes and feeling like a tri-athlete. I made it twenty minutes one day on the treadmill and thought that I had just won the Boston marathon.

We have to start somewhere. Everyone who you see exercising started somewhere. I would wait at the shopping center for a space to open up near the entrance because I had trouble walking to the doors. Just walking from my car was a challenge without getting winded. Remember this: "Just start by moving more today than you did yesterday." Even if you tighten and relax your butt muscles or stretch and move your legs while you are at your desk, that is better than nothing. Tell yourself that today you will take the stairs. The point is that you have to start somewhere and sometime. There is no time better than now. You will be better for it.

I have always said, "The best part of going to the gym is leaving the gym." I still feel this way and probably always will. The first four letters of working out are w-o-r-k. It is easy to not work out. It is easy to make excuses. I made these excuses my whole life, and that's part of the reason why I was in this situation in the first place. It is easy to sit home knowing you should be active. The reality is this: "You have to stay moving to stay alive." You feel so much better when you work out. The sense of accomplishment is so strong after a good workout that it makes you feel great. I always psych myself out knowing that if I use the treadmill four of my workout days that the fifth day will be a great bike ride or an hour of treading water. Treading water is a great and light exercise that can be a deceptively great workout.

I try not to concentrate on time when I am working out. Watch the television when you work out. A good show or movie is always good to pass time. Listen to your favorite music or an audio book. I find staying occupied makes my workout go faster and seem less strenuous. Find out what works best for you to keep you motivated and pass time during your exercise routine.

At this time my cardio is done mostly on the treadmill. I do a 60-minute workout on the treadmill, ten minutes at 3.4 at a 13% incline, then forty minutes at 3.6 to 3.8 and a 13% to 15% incline; then I slowly cool down for ten minutes. I am burning about 1100 – 1180 calories each workout on the treadmill.

I understand that varying the intensity of a workout is also very good for you. I try to mix it up whenever I can. I was never a good runner and never enjoyed it even when I was young and played baseball. Perhaps that will change as I lose more weight and get in even better shape. I said to slowly cool down earlier because I learned it is just as important to cool down as it is to warm up. The heart needs to cool down slowly. In my cardiac rehabilitation after surgery, the nurses would monitor many aspects of my heart rate during exercise. They were able to determine if I was cooling down too fast. Sometimes after a workout they would tell me to drink some water because it must aid in the cool down process somewhat. It is dangerous for you to abruptly stop working out while your heart rate is high.

My exercise workouts always start and end with a good stretching routine. Stretching gets me ready for my workouts. I do several stretches for my back, arms, and legs, holding each stretch for thirty seconds. I learned this from my cardiac rehabilitation. I also like to ride the exercise bicycle or, even better, my hybrid mountain bike outdoors when the weather is nice. I have found a great 60-minute to 70-minute bike route that varies in terrain and intensity near my house. I do enjoy the fresh air. Fresh air is always good.

On Sundays during the summer I was treading water for an hour at the community pool. Try to tread water without touching bottom. I started by only touching bottom four or five times in an hour. I was able to work my way up to not touching bottom for an hour. It became quite challenging and a great fun workout. You will find it to be a workout that is a casual, non-stressful workout, but I felt it really helped my lungs and upper body without much impact. I knew I was burning calories, and it encompassed a little cardio in the routine. I am not a big elliptical or stair-stepper fan, but so many people love it. I say to do what works for you. I often vary my exercise if I am bored or tired. Splitting time between the treadmill and exercise bike is good for me at times.

I try to lift weights on a regular basis. I do about fifteen to twenty repetitions for tone. I use several machines and free weights. Resistance exercise is important for your bones and overall fitness. I am not trying to be Hercules. I just want to feel fit.

I used to go to the gym, and we have all seen the people that seem like they are not working out hard or spend most of their time talking and not working out. I came to realize that no matter what they do, as long as they are doing something, they are benefiting from it. It was good that they just made it to the gym. If you are not exercising at all, then any amount of activity is good for you. I now will take stairs next to the escalator. I get to the top just as fast and feel better for doing so. I don't need to park right next to the front door of a building. In my past, I never would have considered doing these things.

I was at McCarran Airport in Las Vegas recently and flying out of the D gates. If you have ever been there, you would know that there is a rather large escalator leading up to the gates with an equally intimidating set of stairs next to it. I knew I would walk the stairs, and as I was approaching the staircase, behind me was a woman and her child of about ten years old. I could hear the little girl ask her mother if she could walk up the stairs instead of the escalator right next to it. The mother said no, and the child took the escalator. Maybe that mom should have let her kid walk instead of ride the escalator.

Some airports also have long moving flat walkways. I try to walk next to it whenever I can. Anytime I can walk instead of ride, I try to make the choice to walk. At the end of the day, it all adds up.

I try to stay cool when I work out. If I am at home, I can use a fan so I can breathe easier. At a gym it is harder, but you should find a gym near you that has good air circulation. I have left gyms because I couldn't breathe easy in my workouts. I hate a stuffy gym. I know that I will be working up a good sweat, but I just need to be able to breathe easy.

Always check with your doctor before beginning any exercise program. If you are not exercising now, just start somewhere. Put a note in your pocket or put it on your desk at work to remind you to do some sort of exercise.

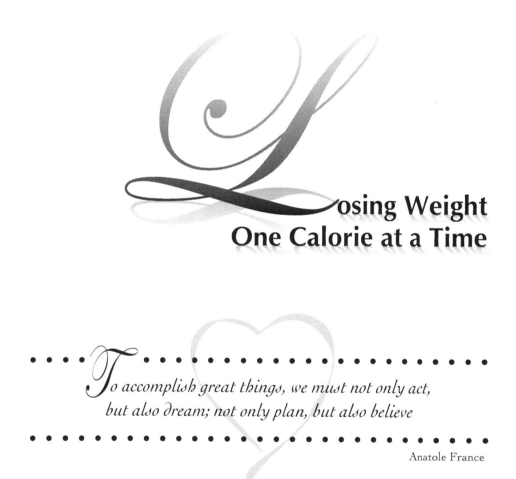

Losing Weight
One Calorie at a Time

To accomplish great things, we must not only act,
but also dream; not only plan, but also believe

Anatole France

The math is easy:

3500 calories is a pound.

Lose 3500 calories and you have lost a pound.

Don't complicate things. Keep it simple. Understand that everything you eat has calories and fat and certain nutritional content. There are websites that show you how many calories you need each day to maintain your current body weight. These sites take into consideration your current height and weight and the amount of daily exercise you do. The amount of exercise is normally listed from sedentary to moderate to extremely active. For example, if you need 2500 calories a day to maintain your current body weight while being extremely active, and you start to eat 2000 calories a day, then after seven days or one week you will have eaten 3500 fewer calories and have lost one pound.

Simple math!

I believe after trying and failing with so many diets over my lifetime that simple common sense will always prevail. You must eat with balance. I try to listen to my body. I feel that my body talks to me sometimes and tells me if I need more sugar or salt. Sometimes I feel I need to eat more fruit. Nutritional balance is a key to any long-term success.

Making the right choices

is the difference, and only we

can make the choices!

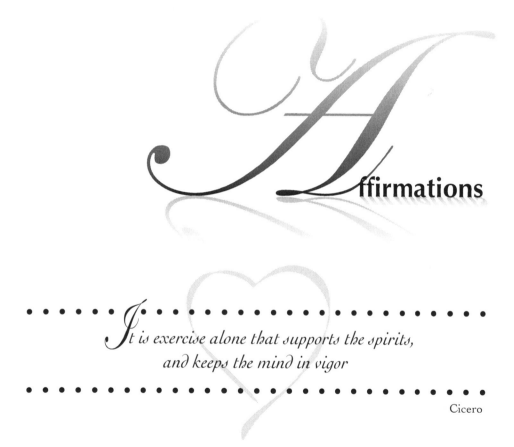

Affirmations

*It is exercise alone that supports the spirits,
and keeps the mind in vigor*

Cicero

I love to keep inspirational notes with little motivational sayings on them around the house and especially on the refrigerator. I keep photos of the big Keith around so that I can see the old me. I will write my next weight loss goal on a sticky note and see it every day. We all like to be inspired by something. Songs are filled with affirmations. Listen to a few of your favorite songs, and they will normally lift you up. I keep photos of myself as a big guy around all the time. My laptop screensaver has a picture of the old me and the new me side by side. I like to show people because they often can't believe it is a picture of me. Anything that motivates and inspires you is a good thing.

Remember...

It's that person you see in the mirror

and old photos who has enabled you

to make a change!

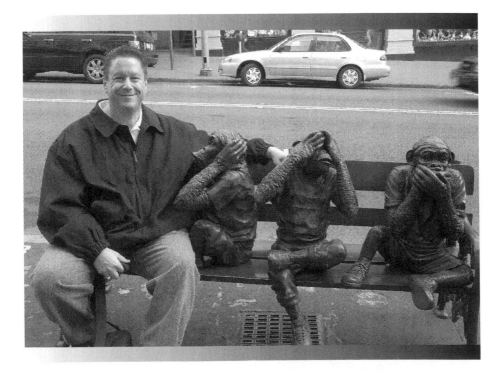

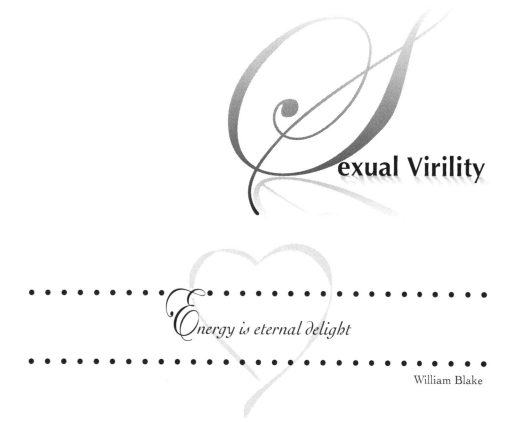

Sexual Virility

Energy is eternal delight

William Blake

I could dedicate a whole book and speak for hours about the change in my sexual "virility" after my heart surgery and subsequent exercise program. Let's put it this way: I am forty-seven years old now and feel eighteen at times. I know that with better circulation from my heart and a good cardio exercise program, my sexual energy is so much better. I feel I had to mention this because it is a part of life. And when life is better, life is good. There are so many studies linking sexual drive to being fit. Having better circulation through a regular cardio exercise program and choosing healthier eating habits...

. . .Can stimulate desires

we thought

were dead or eroded

from our youth!

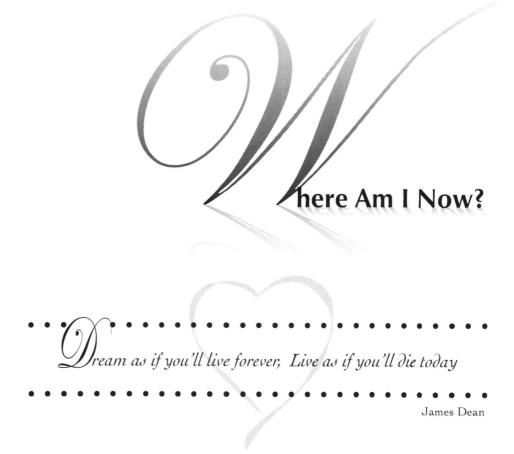

Where Am I Now?

Dream as if you'll live forever, Live as if you'll die today

James Dean

I have been doing rather well both physically and mentally. It has not been easy. The future will not be easy, but nothing in life, it seems, is. I would have done this many years ago if it was easy. My weight is down to **229** from over **414** less than two years ago. That's a 185-pound weight loss without surgery. I wear an extra large dress shirt now and used to wear a 5XL shirt. I even owned a few 6xl shirts. My pants are now a 44 and used to be a snug 60. I know my waist would be smaller if it weren't for the extra fat around my midsection that I am carrying from the weight loss. My blood pressure consistently remains about 120 over 70 or better with a resting pulse rate of 67 to 72. My total cholesterol is about 126 with my LDL (low-density lipoprotein), or bad cholesterol, at 69 and my HDL (high-density lipoprotein), or good cholesterol, at 41. My triglycerides were at 76.

I have been faithfully exercising five to six days a week for at least 60 minutes at a time. I currently take 40 mg of Lipitor®, 81 mg Bayer® baby aspirin, 1000 mg of niacin flush free, and 1200 mg of fish oil three times a day. The Lipitor® is for cholesterol. The baby aspirin is a preventative. The fish oil and niacin and exercise are for my good cholesterol. Lipitor® is the only prescription medication I am on. I am not taking anti-anxiety pills any more. Remember: *Never take any medicines or supplements without consulting your physician first.*

I am trying to eat right, but still find myself wanting to binge on certain foods. I will probably always be a compulsive overeater and need to watch it all the time and be aware of my shortcomings and weaknesses with food. I do find that I am making much better choices for food daily. I have not had the desire for a fast-food hamburger or fries at all. I have somehow managed to stay away from fried chicken and all of the other fast- food nightmares I used to eat all the time. It's just one day at a time.

I want to get down to 214 pounds or under so I can say I lost 200 pounds on my own, an ambitious but, I believe, achievable goal.

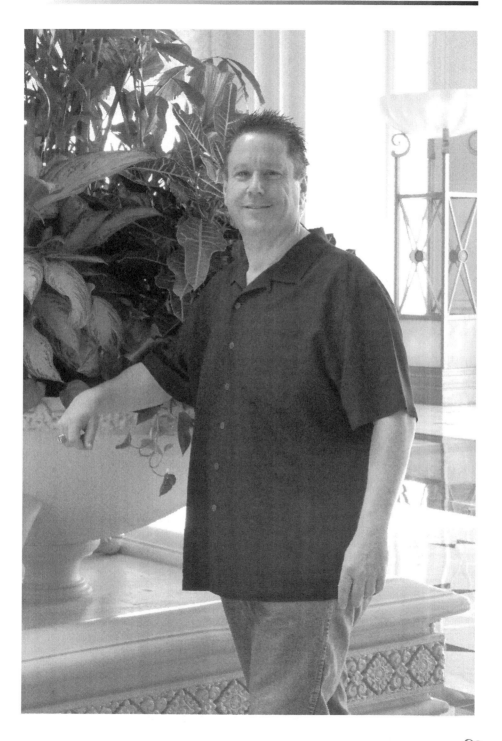

The weight is harder to take off now, and I find it is just as easy to put it back on. When I was 380 pounds, my doctor, Dr. Wikler, asked me what weight I wanted to get down to. I told him 250 pounds. He told me that 210 pounds is a better goal and that 180-190 pounds was optimal. I asked him if he wanted me to cut off my legs. He then asked me if I would rather be fifty or sixty years old and carrying 250 pounds or 210 pounds. I did not need to give him an answer. He saw it on my face. It was a good way to look at it. Ideal weight for my height and bone structure is approximately 185 pounds.

Because I was so big, I am carrying a lot of extra skin around my stomach area. I hate to even talk about it. A while ago, Dr. Wikler brought it up at one of my visits that I will probably need to have some of the extra skin surgically removed at some point. I practically jumped out of the chair and told him I never wanted any more surgery. I think he was surprised by my reaction. He asked me why my reaction was so strong about this topic. I told him I did not want a scar that I could see. He reminded me that I have a 12-inch scar in the middle of my chest. He told me that at some point I would want to consider the surgery if it would give me a better quality of life and make me feel better physically.

The real reason for my reaction, now that I think back on it, is that I was embarrassed that I would even be in the position to have to think of having excess skin removed. He was right. The extra skin is more noticeable to me now. The extra skin also pulls on my back when I try to sleep on my side. It is sometimes uncomfortable. There is a lot of skin in a 400-plus pound body. I will wait until I reach a goal weight to even consider this course of action, but if I stay on the right path, the day will come.

I recently made a surprise visit to my cardiac rehabilitation unit after graduating from the class almost one year ago to the date. I wanted to go for so long but just never got around to it. I wanted to show the nurses and exercise physiologists just how well I was doing.

When I walked into the room, I turned and put a big smile on my face. I stood in the entrance for a moment. The lead nurse, Jackie, and the exercise physiologist, Emily, looked at me. When they realized that it was me they were looking at, their jaws dropped. I had clearly lost a lot of weight and was in much better shape since I saw them a year before when my class ended. I felt like I was seeing family. It was the most encouraging experience I had to date.

We chatted for about twenty minutes, and before I left they told me that I was one of the most successful people they have ever seen go through their program. When I got to the parking lot, my eyes filled with tears because that was one of the biggest, heartfelt compliments I have ever gotten. I realized that I was doing something special. I truly believed that it touched them also to see what their hard work had helped lay the foundation for.

During my most recent routine visit to my cardiologist, I brought Dr. Spaccavento a few pictures of me when I was at least 414 pounds and a picture of me this Christmas holiday at home with my family. Before I went in the room, one of the nurses who had helped me a couple of times in the past looked at me and I said hello with a smile. I know she had no idea who I was because she simply did not recognize me. It wasn't until I got back in the exam room that I asked her if she remembered me, and I showed her the pictures. She was completely blown away. When I met with the doctor, I could tell how proud he was of me and that a patient of his was doing what the patient should be doing to live a long, heart-healthy life.

When I left the examination room to schedule my next appointment with him, the scheduler did not recognize me. When she realized that it was me in front of her after I gave her my name, she smiled from ear to ear. She told me that she had thought I was a new patient. The office manager saw this and after realizing that it was me came out from her desk and gave me a big hug.

When I have had to show my drivers license for identification in the states or present my passport when I travel, there have been several times when the person looking at my old picture gives me a great compliment. The best was a Chinese immigration officer who had to take three takes on my photograph. She couldn't believe how much weight I had lost. She told me to keep up the good work. She barely spoke any English. It sure put a smile on my face.

Every time I go to my regular doctor's office and see Dr. Eric for my routine exam and blood work, I get so encouraged. Dr. Eric is the best, and I credit him with saving my life. He was, after all, the doctor who initially saw that something was wrong and steered me on the right path. He is always impressed with my determination to change my life and to be physically fit. He has been with me every step of the way.

My family has been so supportive. My brothers and sisters have been so encouraging. They have been my biggest cheerleaders. My nieces and nephews give me purpose and headaches. They are the children I never had. I thank my brothers and sisters for sharing them with me. I live for my family. I love them so much. I have so many close friends. I am so lucky. One thing my sister Candy commented on when she was taking care of me was the number of friends and people that really seemed to care about me. She was amazed at how many close friends I have.

My friends have been so supportive. I find so many things every day in so many ways that inspire me. Little things I do or see give me such great inspiration and motivation. My mother, Joan; my father, Mike; my aunt, Anneta; and my beloved sister Stacy have passed away.

*N**ot a day goes by*

that I don't talk to them

in spirit!

I know that they see me and are with me with each step I take on the treadmill and with each pound of weight I lose.

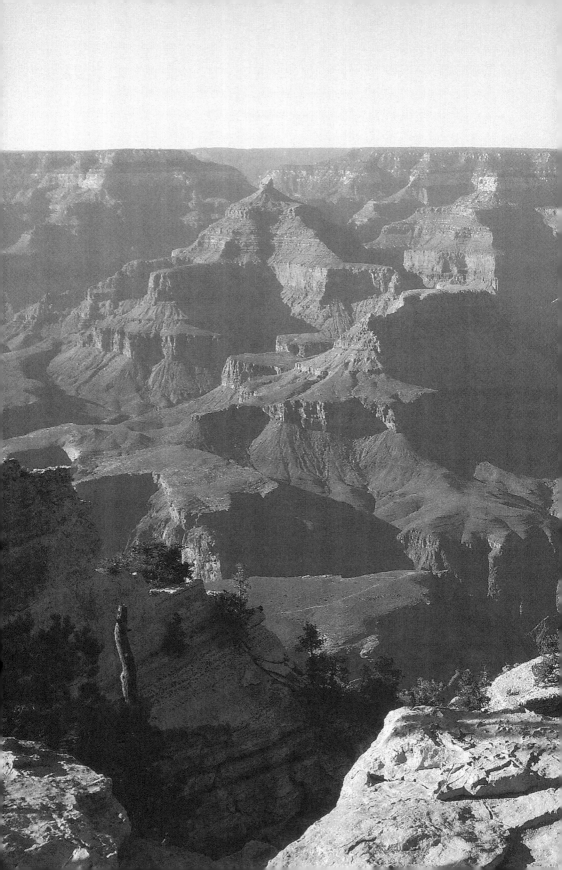

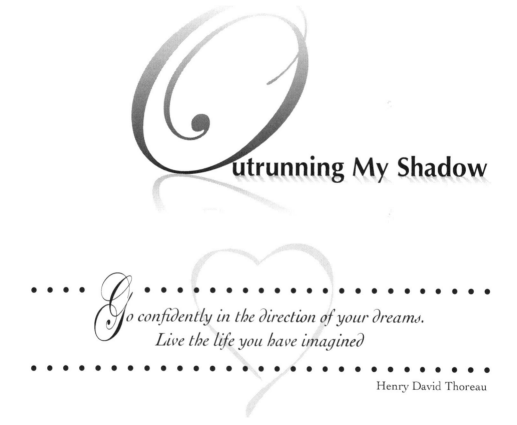

Outrunning My Shadow

Go confidently in the direction of your dreams.
Live the life you have imagined

Henry David Thoreau

A lot of my friends have asked me how I came up with the name for my book. The name came to me one night at 3:00 a.m. in my sleep. I remember waking up and scratching it down on a piece of paper that I kept next to my bed. I had recently taken a couple days off and drove to the Grand Canyon and Sedona, Arizona. While at the Grand Canyon I walked a few miles along the southern rim. It was late in the afternoon, and I remembered all the people that were there to see the sunset. If you haven't been to the Grand Canyon, let me tell you that it is one of the most majestic places on earth. It will truly take your breath away. Seeing the sun set in the Canyon is spectacular to say the least. It seems as if a million colors and shadows come to life and the Canyon relaxes before it goes to sleep and dreams for the night.

I started my walk to the west toward the sun, which was getting lower on the horizon along the rim. After a couple miles, I turned around to walk back. I was now heading east walking away from the sun. My shadow was in front of me now. It was getting longer as the sun was getting lower on the horizon behind me. My shadow was getting so much longer that it seemed as though it was leading my way and pointing me along the path with every footstep.

I kept walking towards my shadow. I had wondered,

"If I was walking away from the sun, was I now walking into the sunset?"

It then dawned on me,

"Sometimes you need to walk away from something to see what's in front of you."

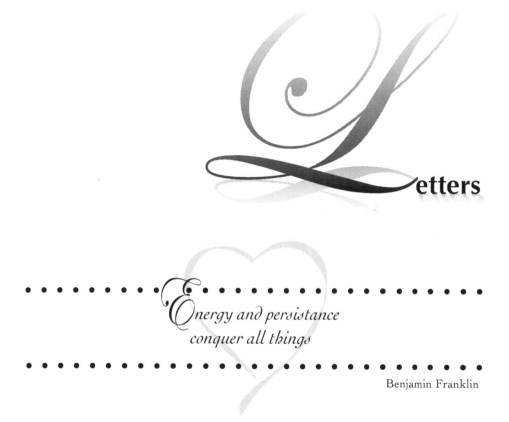

*L*etters

These are just some of the notes I got by email from a few of my friends after I let them know what was going on. In addition, I have shown some of the correspondence I sent to Dr. Hirsch keeping him posted. I received so many cards and well wishes from friends and family. It was so nice knowing so many people cared.

Keith,

I just want to say "thank you" for sharing this with me. I don't remember if I told you about losing my brother last year, but he didn't have the 2ND chance you are getting; his blockage happened so fast.....there was nothing that could have been done. I have to tell you that I am a little shocked (but not totally) to hear about your condition......

I have a very good friend that is a 30yr RN and Cardiac Specialist at Long Beach Memorial. She and I talked at length about the information you shared with me. She is so positive about your future and how happy your heart is going to be with "new pipes"! Of course you'll have to change some habits..... Jen says "He'll be amazed (almost immediately) at how good His body is going to feel with all that blood and oxygen flowing and being forced into His extremities." She called it "a new life"! I am really looking forward to hearing about it from you Keith.

I understand that when the procedure is

complete you'll be quite literally "back on your feet" within a day or two, that's amazing!

Keith, what is your birth date? I just had my 51st on the 18th of July (the day you met with Dr. Spaccavento).

I don't really have any (male) friends that I care about since losing my Brother and Father last year, so I guess you're it! LOL Too bad for you Bro.....
Anyway, I'll be back in the States shortly and will come to visit....You may or may not have had the procedure by then, if you have you'll need some weeks away from everything and everyone I'm sure.

Keith, please let me know when and where you decide to have the procedure......I may not be able to be there, but I can send a lot of positive energy your way.

I sure am looking forward to riding with you again,

Mark
Camp Taji, Iraq
APO AE

Boom Boom,

I am so glad to see that your attitude is so positive. It can be so easy to just give up. Please don't do that. Keep up the healthy diet and the walking. It's so important that you keep up the changes in your habits. We need your shit grin around for a little while. You never know when a guy with my personality may need a reference, not that I am one to ever lose my cool or scream and yell or anything like that. You know how smooth and under control I am. Just like that time I nicely asked that guy to kindly leave our lot that one morning me and you were at the desk. (Remember that? I loved that one.) Just kidding. I have matured if you can believe it.

Anyway, Bro, Please take good care of yourself and keep me posted. I should be in town in a few weeks and would love to take you to a nice dinner at Morton's or somewhere nice. I'll keep in touch and keep up the positive attitude.

Harley

Well, I'm at a loss as to something clever to say. Thanks for sharing the news. Time to get serious and get stuff straightened out. I'm sure your docs have given you direction on diet and activity; if not, let me know and I'll find a cardio guy here and get you whatever you need. Surgery will be a bitch, but doable. I'm sure you've thought about things, but now is an equally good time to think about what you plan to do with the rest of your life. A little heart thing to deal with now, but then another 40 to 50 years. Maybe it's time to change locale and lifestyle. Let me know if you'd like to do something together out here. I think there are some good opportunities with the base realignment bringing 10,000 soldiers to Ft Meade and Aberdeen.

I have the family in Hawaii for a two-week vacation. I'm not sure what 2008 will bring for me and the company. I'm still kind of burnt out. I'm hoping the islands recharge me.

If you need me to come out to help with anything or if I can do anything for the family here, call my cell and I'll be there.

Talk to you.
Love you brother. Be strong.
Brad

Damn my brother that is a lot to go through, but the Fox Run Boyz are a tough crew. If there is anything I can do for you please let me know. You are in our thoughts and we are always here for you. My cell phone number is 941-***-****. Call anytime.

Dave

Letter to:
Glen Hirsch, MD Johns Hopkins Cardiology

July 18ᵗʰ, 2007

Hi Glen, Hope all is well.

I met with my regular doctor, Eric Wikler yesterday and with my cardiologist, Leo J. Spaccavento today. Wikler reviewed my latest lab results. All looked good he said except my good cholesterol was low. My BP yesterday was 120 over 76 and today it was 120 over 80. My weight was 371 today.

I have asked Spaccavento's office to forward all of my stuff to you. He will be sending you all of the things that you requested and all of the things on the Cleveland clinic checklist. I am obtaining a second opinion from the Cleveland clinic. They do an e-Consult. I will let you know and forward you all of the Cleveland stuff when available. Let me know if anything you need is missing and I will get on it fast.

Spaccavento told me the baby aspirin was good. He also put me on Plavix® 75mg, one a day, up until 1 week before my surgery. I am still on the Lipitor® 20mg.

FYI below is the problem as I know it that I sent to Cleveland clinic so it will give you an idea refresher of what's up again.

What is the primary (chief) problem for which you are seeking this second opinion consultation?

I had an angiogram on July 6, 2007, and was told that I had all three major arteries completely blocked and there may be more blockage. I was told I need bypass surgery but because of my weight on the 6th of 380 pounds the cardiac surgeon on call decided that due to what I am assuming were my vital signs he felt that I should wait until my weight got down to 300 pounds before surgery. Dr. Spaccavento told me my heart was strong and that an army of collateral veins or arteries over the years has taken over the blood and oxygen supply to my heart. I meet with Dr. Spaccavento on July 18th and will learn more after the hospital visit and angiogram. In the 2 months prior to my angiogram I had gone from 414 lbs to 380 the day of the angiogram. My blood pressure was normal and my cholesterol had come down to 149 I believe. For two months I had been eating a very low fat diet and walking on my treadmill. I had worked up to about 22 minutes at a distance of 3/4 to .8 of a mile. I felt really good. The last time I walked was the night before the angiogram. I felt I was doing all the right things. This is my story that led up to the angiogram. About 3 months ago I got lightheaded three times in a period of one week. On a scale of 1-10, 10 being passed out I would say I had a 6, a 7.5 and a 9. After the nine I decided to go see a doctor for a physical which I had not had in years. It is important to note I have not had any more lightheadedness. I saw Eric Wikler, D.O., Wikler family practice 702-***-****. He ordered blood work and the results just showed high cholesterol. He prescribed Lipitor® and I continue to take it today. All of my other stuff came back ok. he did an EKG and an abnormality showed up and he told me a stress test would be warranted. He referred me to Dr. Spaccavento and we did the nuclear stress test without the treadmill, i.e., me lying on my back and they gave me the IV that raced my heart. The results I believe showed signs of a possible blockage on an artery. Dr. Spaccavento then thought an angiogram was in order. At the angiogram I believe he was quite surprised to find the extent of blockage that he found. Now I need more guidance. Please help.

What is the patient's medical diagnosis?

How long can I wait for the surgery and is it necessary? Should I be waiting until I get to 300 pounds or lower? I understand that if I get signs I need to call 911. I am not stupid.

Glen, thanks so much. I have learned that the stress test showed some more stuff than what I thought.

I will keep you posted of any changes. I meet with a surgeon for another opinion in a week or two out here.

Call me if you need any more information at all.
702-***-****

With great respect and gratitude,

Keith

August 8, 2007

Hi Glen,

Here is the latest news. I met with the two surgeons. V.C. Smith last night and Dr. Wiencek this morning. Both said the surgery should be done at the earliest possible time. They both said the surgery can be done as safely as possible, even though my weight is high. They both felt the risk of waiting far outweighed the risk of doing the procedure soon. Both of the doctors were great and it was comforting to me and my sister, who came with me, that I could have two great choices of doctors. I believe the surgery will be in two to three weeks. I am going to use Dr. V.C. Smith I believe. He is head of the unit at St. Rose hospital in Henderson.

Dr. Wiencek did mention to us that he would do an "OFF PUMP CORONARY BYPASS SURGERY." I did not clarify with V.C. Smith if he would use that procedure. If he does not, should I reconsider Dr. Wiencek as the surgeon? What do you think? I will call Smiths office and ask them tomorrow and get the answer of the exact procedure.
I will keep you posted.

Thank you again for all your help.
Keith

Letter to:
 "my friends before my surgery"

August 10, 2007

   Hi everyone. Hope you are doing well. I just
wanted to give everyone an update on the latest news.
   All of the opinions that I have received after
the angiogram on July 6th, with the exception of
one, have advised me to have the surgery sooner
than later. Johns Hopkins, Cleveland Clinic, and three
cardiologists and three surgeons all agreed that
the risk to wait far outweighed the risk to do the
surgery now. I received a total of eight professional
opinions and due to the severity and complexity of
the problem the time is now.
   The positive news is that all of my vitals are
excellent. With the exception of my weight and my
heart right now I am in unusually good health. I
have been doing real well on the weight issue also.
If things go well within the first 5-8 days during
and after surgery, I should be on the road to a great
recovery and hopefully a long and healthy life.
   Candy and I interviewed and met with the two
top coronary heart surgeons here in Las Vegas. Both
surgeons were outstanding and the choice was made
more difficult by the fact that we very much liked

them both. I picked Dr. V.C. Smith. He is supposed to be an outstanding surgeon.

My surgery is scheduled for August 23 at St Rose Sienna Hospital here in Henderson. Dr. Smith is chief of the Cardiac Unit and it is supposed to be top notch with an outstanding critical care unit.

Although I am needless to say a little freaked out about the situation, as I have told many of you, better this be me than my nieces, nephews, brothers, sisters, family or my friends that I love. I really mean that. Candy has been a huge support for me being here. She is like a pit bull when it comes to these doctors and getting the correct information. Besides all that, I know that I have not one but two guardian angels to make sure things are ok.

I will try to keep everyone posted if there are any changes in the schedule. When I am in the hospital Candy's cell phone number is 1-434-***-****. If she does not answer, leave her a message and she will call you back. I don't think they allow me to use my cell phone in the ICU while I have a breathing tube shoved down my throat. Just kidding. Wish me luck and always remember to do something good for someone else.

Love, Keith

September 13, 2007

Hi Dr. Glen,

I survived. Thanks so much for all your guidance through this ordeal. I know Candy, my sister, spoke with you after surgery. It has been 21 days so far. It's been a bitch but I have had a lot of help and support. I don't know how people go through this without the help I have had. Candy has been here the whole time and has literally waited on me hand and foot. I have been feeling a little better each day. It still hurts a lot but I know that will pass as time goes on. The surgeon said the bypasses were successful.

I have been resting a lot and healing and have started walking slowly for 15 minutes 3 times a day. I am down to 325 from 414 on April 9th. Eating 3 to 4 times a day. I eat a lot of proteins and carbohydrates, keeping it low in fat and low in calories. Pretty well balanced with all the food groups.

Thanks again for all your help. Sorry it took me so long to give you an update but I just got back on the computer.

With the greatest respect and heartfelt appreciation,

Keith

Letter to:
"my friends and family"

September 23, 2007

I am doing better the last two days. It has been 4 weeks out of surgery and I am making progress. The pain has settled a lot. Don't get me wrong, it still hurts but not as bad. I have been walking almost every day. Today I walked around the block about 22 minutes at an ok pace. I want to go back to work real bad. Tomorrow I am going to attempt to go in for a couple hours I hope. It is all feel at this point while I must keep in mind the sternum takes 6-7 weeks to heal and protect it. I am down to 319 pounds from 414 on April 9th. I am trying to do all the right things, diet, rest etc....

I start cardiac rehab in 2 weeks (they must allow 6 weeks for the sternum bone to heal). It will be good for me. It is 3 times a week for an hour. At least I think it will keep me focused on doing all the things I have been doing.

Candy has been an unbelievable help. I can't tell anyone how much she has done for me. I never could have done this alone. She has not complained once, even when I act like an ass.

Thanks for keeping me in your thoughts

Love
Keith

February 10, 2008

Hi Glen,

I hope this note finds you in good health and happiness.

I just wanted to update you on my progress so far. I am down to 273 from 414 last May. I exercise everyday for cardio. It is no problem for me to walk for 60 minutes at 3.2 speed at 7% incline. I try to get in my cardio zone of 124 – 130 heart rate on my stationary bike and treadmill. I just purchased a new bicycle that I rode to work yesterday. The bike will add to my physical fitness regimen a few times a month. I am trying to mix it up and keep it fun. I am eating a low fat and low calorie diet. I splurge not often but don't deny myself when I need to reward myself. I have had red meat probably only 10 or 11 times since last May. A lot of chicken in my diet.

I do feel some discomfort every once in a while in the sternum still but my cardiologist told me to give it a year. The healing takes a while I guess from open heart.

My latest lab results from my regular Dr. visit two weeks ago are as follows:

136 total cholesterol

LDL 96

HDL 29 – I have been taking fish oil 1000mg and just started on Niacin flush free 500 mg a day to see if I can elevate my HDL. My regular doctor wants me to try this for 3 months.

Triglycerides – 85

Blood pressure is in totally excellent range.

Medicines are:

Lipitor® 20mg – 1 a day at night

Baby aspirin – 1 a day at night

Fish oil 1000mg – 3 times daily

Niacin – 500mg flush free – 1 a day at night

Xanax® – .5 mg – occasionally I will take Xanax®.

I still have trouble sleeping now and then and do believe it is 100% anxiety. Family and work seem to be the hot buttons of restlessness. I do love my family and love my job also. I am a very lucky guy.

I go back to my regular doctor at the end of April for my annual physical. I trust all will be o.k. I assume he will do a routine EKG, the same one that saw the abnormality last April. I am not sure when a nuclear treadmill stress test is given or when I get my heart looked at again; but, my cardiologist did indicate it was within a couple of years.

I plan on going to Hong Kong in the middle of April. I guess it has always been on my "bucket list."

Take care, I will keep you posted. I wanted to share with you my progress and let you know I am still very motivated. The goal is to be at 210lbs. God willing one day at a time I can do the right things to get there.

Thanks for everything,
I will stay in touch.
Keith

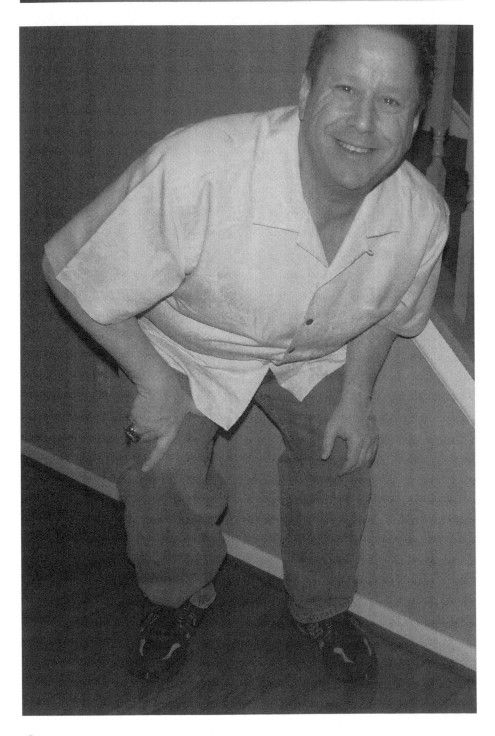

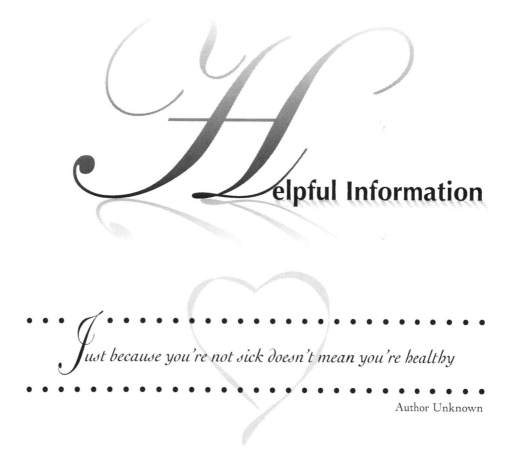

Helpful Information

Just because you're not sick doesn't mean you're healthy

Author Unknown

The following information should give you some guidance and put some of the numbers and terminology in perspective. Your doctor will be able to summarize your results and should be able to give you good advice and direction. Remember that your numbers may be different due to medication or other medical or physical issues, which you should always discuss with your doctor.

The following is reprinted by permission from the National Institutes of Health, National Heart Lung Blood Institute, a division of The Department of Health and Human Services website.

Anatomy of the Heart

Your heart is located under the ribcage in the center of your chest between your right and left lung. It's shaped like an upside-down pear. Its muscular walls beat, or contract, pumping blood continuously to all parts of your body.

The size of your heart can vary depending on your age, size, or the condition of your heart. A normal, healthy, adult heart most often is the size of an average clenched adult fist. Some diseases of the heart can cause it to become larger.

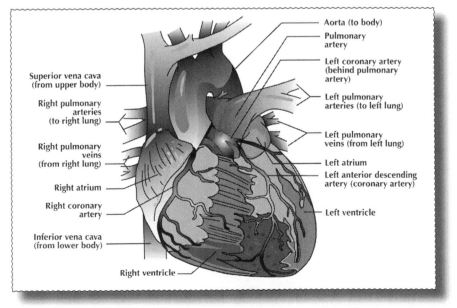

Illustration: Outside of a normal, healthy, human heart

The illustration shows the front surface of the heart, including the coronary arteries and major blood vessels.

The heart is the muscle in the lower half of the picture. The heart has four chambers. The right and left atria (AY-tree-uh) are shown in purple. The right and left ventricles (VEN-trih-kuls) are shown in dark grey.

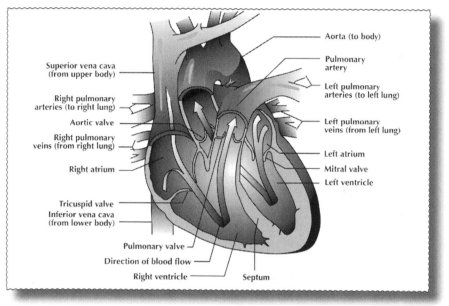

Illustration: Inside of a normal, healthy, human heart

The picture shows the inside of your heart and how it's divided into four chambers. The two upper chambers of your heart are called atria. The atria receive and collect blood. The two lower chambers of your heart are called ventricles. The ventricles pump blood out of your heart into the circulatory system to other parts of your body.

What Is Coronary Heart Disease?

Heart disease is caused by narrowing of the coronary arteries that feed the heart. Like any muscle, the heart needs a constant supply of oxygen and nutrients, which are carried to it by the blood in the coronary arteries. When the coronary arteries become narrowed or clogged by cholesterol and fat deposits—a process called atherosclerosis—and cannot supply enough blood to the heart, the result is

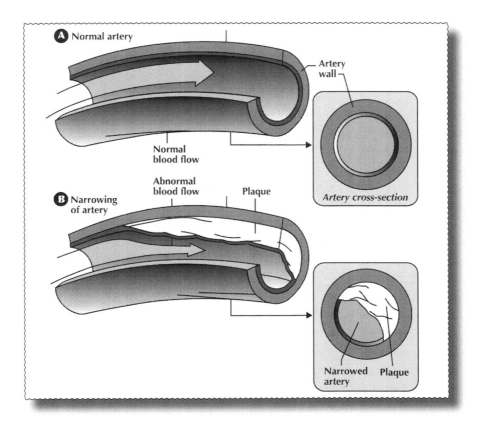

coronary heart disease (CHD). If not enough oxygen-carrying blood reaches the heart, you may experience chest pain called angina. If the blood supply to a portion of the heart is completely cut off by total blockage of a coronary artery, the result is a heart attack. This is usually due to a sudden closure from a blood clot forming on top of a previous narrowing.

Cholesterol is a waxy, fat-like substance that occurs naturally in all parts of the body and that your body needs to function normally. It is present in cell walls or membranes everywhere in the body, including the brain, nerves, muscle, skin, liver, intestines, and heart. Your body uses cholesterol to produce many hormones, vitamin D, and the bile acids that help to digest fat. It takes only a small amount of cholesterol in the blood to meet these needs. If you have too much cholesterol in your bloodstream, the excess is deposited in arteries, including the coronary arteries, where it contributes to the narrowing and blockages that cause the signs and symptoms of heart disease.

What Is a Heart Attack?

A heart attack occurs when blood flow to a section of heart muscle becomes blocked. If the flow of blood isn't restored quickly, the section of heart muscle becomes damaged from lack of oxygen and begins to die.

Heart attack is a leading killer of both men and women in the United States. But fortunately, today there are excellent treatments for heart attack that can save lives and prevent disabilities. Treatment is most effective when started within 1 hour of the beginning of symptoms. If you think you or someone you're with is having a heart attack, call 9–1–1 right away.

Overview

Heart attacks occur most often as a result of a condition called coronary artery disease (CAD). In CAD, a fatty material called plaque (plak) builds up over many years on the inside walls of the coronary arteries (the arteries that supply blood and oxygen to your heart). Eventually, an area of plaque can rupture, causing a blood clot to form on the surface of the plaque. If the clot becomes large enough, it can mostly or completely block the flow of oxygen-rich blood to the part of the heart muscle fed by the artery.

Heart With Muscle Damage and a Blocked Artery

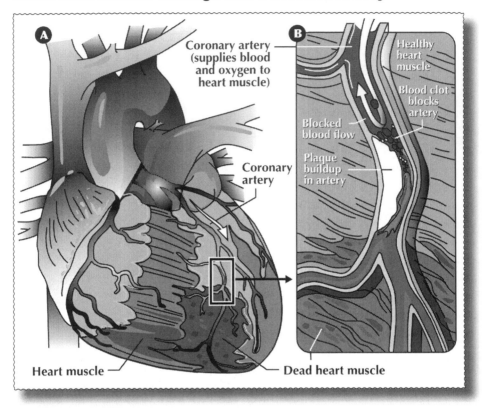

Figure A is an overview of a heart and coronary artery showing damage (dead heart muscle) caused by a heart attack. Figure B is a cross-section of the coronary artery with plaque buildup and a blood clot.

During a heart attack, if the blockage in the coronary artery isn't treated quickly, the heart muscle will begin to die and be replaced by scar tissue. This heart damage may not be obvious, or it may cause severe or long-lasting problems.

Severe problems linked to heart attack can include **heart failure** and life-threatening **arrhythmias** (irregular heartbeats). Heart failure is a condition in which the heart can't pump enough blood throughout the body. Ventricular fibrillation is a serious arrhythmia that can cause death if not treated quickly.

The most common heart attack signs and symptoms are:

Chest discomfort or pain, uncomfortable pressure, squeezing, fullness, or pain in the center of the chest that can be mild or strong. This discomfort or pain lasts more than a few minutes or goes away and comes back.
Upper body discomfort in one or both arms, the back, neck, jaw, or stomach.
Pain that spreads from the chest to the shoulders, jaw, or arms.
Shortness of breath may occur with or before chest discomfort.
Chest discomfort with lightheadedness, fainting, sweating, nausea, or shortness of breath.
Other signs include nausea (feeling sick to your stomach), vomiting, lightheadedness or fainting, or breaking out in a cold sweat.

If you think you or someone you know may be having a heart attack:

Call 9–1–1 within a few minutes — 5 at the most — of the start of symptoms.
If your symptoms stop completely in less than 5 minutes, still call your doctor.
Only take an ambulance to the hospital. Going in a private car can delay treatment.
Take a nitroglycerin pill if your doctor has prescribed this type of medicine.

What if I have the warning signs of a heart attack?

You should know the symptoms of a heart attack so that you can get immediate medical help.

Get . . . Help . . . Quickly!

Acting fast at the first sign of heart attack symptoms can save your life and limit damage to your heart. Treatment is most effective when started within 1 hour of the beginning of symptoms.

These symptoms may be severe from the start, or they may be mild at first, then gradually worsen. In some people, the warning symptoms come and go.

If you experience any symptoms of a heart attack, get medical help immediately. Be sure you know the phone number so you can get emergency transportation to the hospital. If you are having a heart attack, getting to the hospital fast is very important. Medical treatment, including clot-dissolving medicine, can save lives and reduce damage to the heart muscle, but only if it is started very soon after a heart attack occurs.

Talk with your doctor about the symptoms of a heart attack and what to do if you experience them.

Outlook

Each year, about 1.1 million people in the United States have heart attacks, and almost half of them die. CAD, which often results in a heart attack, is the leading killer of both men and women in the United States.

Many more people could recover from heart attacks if they got help faster. Of the people who die from heart attacks, about half die within an hour of the first symptoms and before they reach the hospital.

What Is an Electrocardiogram?

An electrocardiogram (e-lek-tro-KAR-de-o-gram), or EKG, is a simple, painless test that records the heart's electrical activity. To understand this test, it helps to understand how the heart works.

With each heartbeat, an electrical signal spreads from the top of the heart to the bottom. As it travels, the signal causes the heart to contract and pump blood. The process repeats with each new heartbeat. The heart's electrical signals set the rhythm of the heartbeat.

WHAT AN ELECTROCARDIOGRAM (EKG) TEST SHOWS
How fast your heart is beating
Whether the rhythm of your heartbeat is steady or irregular
The strength and timing of electrical signals as they pass through each part of your heart
This test is used to detect and evaluate many heart problems, such as heart attack, arrhythmia (ah-RITH-me-ah), and heart failure. EKG results also can suggest other disorders that affect heart function.
EKGs also are used to monitor how the heart is working.

What Is a Nuclear Heart Scan?

A nuclear heart scan is a type of medical test that allows your doctor to get important information about the health of your heart. During a nuclear heart scan, a safe, radioactive material called a tracer is injected through a vein into your bloodstream. The tracer then travels to your heart. The tracer releases energy, which special cameras outside of your body detect. The cameras use the energy to create pictures of different parts of your heart.

NUCLEAR HEART SCANS ARE USED FOR THREE MAIN PURPOSES

To provide information about the flow of blood throughout the heart muscle. If the scan shows that one part of the heart muscle isn't receiving blood, it's a sign of a possible narrowing or blockage in the coronary arteries (the arteries that supply blood and oxygen to your heart). Decreased blood flow through the coronary arteries may mean you have coronary artery disease (CAD). CAD can lead to angina, heart attack, and other heart problems. When a nuclear heart scan is performed for this purpose, it's called myocardial perfusion scanning.

To look for damaged heart muscle. Damage may be due to a previous heart attack, injury, infection, or medicine. When a nuclear heart scan is performed for this purpose, it's called myocardial viability testing.

To see how well your heart pumps blood out to your body. When a nuclear heart scan is performed for this purpose, it's called ventricular function scanning.

Usually, two sets of pictures are taken during a nuclear heart scan. The first set is taken when the heart is beating fast due to you exercising. This is called a cardiac stress test. If you can't exercise, your heart rate can be increased using medicines such as adenosine, dipyridamole, or dobutamine.

The second set of pictures is taken later, when the heart is at rest and beating at a normal rate.

Helpful Hints To Monitor Your New Lifestyle

1. Record your test results at each visit.

2. Set realistic short-term goals and write them down.

3. Review your goals during each visit with your health care provider.

4. Share your goals with your family and friends. Support is often the key to success.

If you find yourself unable to keep to your plan, write down all of the reasons that you think are responsible. Next, write down what alternatives you have if that situation happens again. If you prepare an alternate strategy in advance, you are more likely to stick to your plan and reach your goals.

What Is Cardiac Catheterization?

Cardiac catheterization (KATH-e-ter-i-ZA-shun) is a medical procedure used to diagnose and treat certain heart conditions. A long, thin, flexible tube called a catheter is put into a blood vessel in your arm, groin (upper thigh), or neck and threaded to your heart. Through the catheter, doctors can perform diagnostic tests and treatments on your heart.

Sometimes a special dye is put into the catheter to make the insides of your heart and blood vessels show up on x rays. The dye can show whether a material called plaque (plak) has narrowed or blocked any of your heart's arteries (called coronary arteries).

Plaque is made up of fat, cholesterol, calcium, and other substances found in your blood. The buildup of plaque narrows the inside of the arteries and, in time, may restrict blood flow to your heart. When this happens, it's called coronary artery disease (CAD).

Blockages in the arteries also can be seen using ultrasound during cardiac catheterization. Ultrasound uses sound waves to create detailed pictures of the heart's blood vessels.

Doctors may take samples of blood and heart muscle during cardiac catheterization, as well as do minor heart surgery.

Cardiologists (doctors who specialize in treating people who have heart problems) usually perform cardiac catheterization in a hospital. You're awake during the procedure, and it causes little to no pain, although you may feel some soreness in the blood vessel where your doctor put the catheter. Cardiac catheterization rarely causes serious complications.

Cholesterol levels

"When I have my cholesterol checked, there are three critical numbers that are important to me. Your doctor will help you evaluate your numbers with you. The three things that I check regularly are my total cholesterol, my good cholesterol or HDL, and my bad cholesterol or LDL. I found out that having your good cholesterol levels too low is just as dangerous as having high bad cholesterol."

TOTAL CHOLESTEROL LEVEL
Less than 200 is best.
200 to 239 is borderline high.
240 or more means you're at increased risk for heart disease.

LDL OR "BAD" CHOLESTEROL LEVELS
Below 100 is ideal for people who have a higher risk of heart disease.
100 to 129 is near optimal.
130 to 159 is borderline high.
160 or more means you're at a higher risk for heart disease.

HDL OR "GOOD" CHOLESTEROL LEVELS
Less than 40 means you're at higher risk for heart disease.
60 or higher greatly reduces your risk of heart disease.

"The doctors believe that my having very low good cholesterol (HDL) for so many years was a major factor in my coronary artery disease. Perhaps genetics played a part in this also. My good cholesterol is now in the normal range. A friend of mine told me that an easy way to remember which is good and bad is that the LDL or bad cholesterol begin with the letter "L" for lethal. It really is amazing how you can effect and improve your own numbers over time with regular exercise, healthy eating, and medication, if necessary."

What Is Cholesterol?

To understand high blood cholesterol (ko-LES-ter-ol), it is important to know more about cholesterol.

Cholesterol is a waxy, fat-like substance that is found in all cells of the body. Your body needs some cholesterol to work the right way. Your body makes all the cholesterol it needs.

Cholesterol is also found in some of the foods you eat.

Your body uses cholesterol to make hormones, vitamin D, and substances that help you digest foods.

Blood is watery, and cholesterol is fatty. Just like oil and water, the two do not mix. To travel in the bloodstream, cholesterol is carried in small packages called lipoproteins (lip-o-PRO-teens). The small packages are made of fat (lipid) on the inside and proteins on the outside. Two kinds of lipoproteins carry cholesterol throughout your body. It is important to have healthy levels of both:

Low-density lipoprotein (LDL) cholesterol is sometimes called bad cholesterol.

High LDL cholesterol leads to a buildup of cholesterol in arteries. The higher the LDL level in your blood, the greater chance you have of getting heart disease.

High-density lipoprotein (HDL) cholesterol is sometimes called good cholesterol.

HDL carries cholesterol from other parts of your body back to your liver. The liver removes the cholesterol from your body. The higher your HDL cholesterol level, the lower your chance of getting heart disease.

What Is High Blood Cholesterol?

Too much cholesterol in the blood, or high blood cholesterol, can be serious. People with high blood cholesterol have a greater chance of getting heart disease. High blood cholesterol on its own does not cause symptoms, so many people are unaware that their cholesterol level is too high.

Cholesterol can build up in the walls of your arteries (blood vessels that carry blood from the heart to other parts of the body). This buildup of cholesterol is called plaque (plak). Over time, plaque can cause narrowing of the arteries. This is called atherosclerosis (ath-er-o-skler-O-sis), or hardening of the arteries.

Special arteries, called coronary arteries, bring blood to the heart. Narrowing of your coronary arteries due to plaque can stop or slow down the flow of blood to your heart. When the arteries narrow, the amount of oxygen-rich blood is decreased. This is called coronary heart disease (CHD). Large plaque areas can lead to chest pain called angina (an-JI-nuh or AN-juh-nuh). Angina happens when the heart does not receive enough oxygen-rich blood. Angina is a common symptom of CHD.

Some plaques have a thin covering and can burst (rupture), releasing cholesterol and fat into the bloodstream. The release of cholesterol and fat may cause your blood to clot. A clot can block the flow of blood. This blockage can cause angina or a heart attack.

Lowering your cholesterol level decreases your chance for having a plaque burst and cause a heart attack. Lowering cholesterol may also slow down, reduce, or even stop plaque from building up.

Plaque and resulting health problems can also occur in arteries elsewhere in the body.

Triglycerides

Triglycerides are a form of fat carried through the bloodstream. Most of your body's fat is in the form of triglycerides stored in fat tissue. Only a small portion of your triglycerides is found in the bloodstream. High blood triglyceride levels alone do not necessarily cause atherosclerosis (the buildup of cholesterol and fat in the walls of arteries). But some lipoproteins that are rich in triglycerides also contain cholesterol, which causes atherosclerosis in some people with high triglycerides, and high triglycerides are often accompanied by other factors (such as low HDL or a tendency toward diabetes) that raise heart disease risk. So high triglycerides may be a sign of a lipoprotein problem that contributes to heart disease.

TRIGLYCERIDE LEVELS	
Normal	Less than 150 mg/dL
Borderline-high	150-199 mg/dL
High	200-499 mg/dL
Very High	500 mg/dL or above

What Is High Blood Pressure?

High blood pressure (HBP) is a serious condition that can lead to <u>coronary heart disease, heart failure, stroke, kidney failure</u>, and other health problems.

"Blood pressure" is the force of blood pushing against the walls of the arteries as the heart pumps out blood. If this pressure rises and stays high over time, it can damage the body in many ways.

Overview

About 1 in 3 adults in the United States has HBP. HBP itself usually has no symptoms. You can have it for years without knowing it. During this time, though, it can damage the heart, blood vessels, kidneys, and other parts of your body.

This is why knowing your blood pressure numbers is important, even when you're feeling fine. If your blood pressure is normal, you can work with your health care team to keep it that way. If your blood pressure is too high, you need treatment to prevent damage to your body's organs.

Blood Pressure Numbers

Blood pressure numbers include systolic (sis-TOL-ik) and diastolic (di-a-STOL-ik) pressures. Systolic blood pressure is the pressure when the heart beats while pumping blood. Diastolic blood pressure is the pressure when the heart is at rest between beats.

You will most often see blood pressure numbers written with the systolic number above or before the diastolic, such as 120/80 mmHg. (The mmHg is millimeters of mercury – the units used to measure blood pressure.)

The table below shows normal numbers for adults. It also shows which numbers put you at greater risk for health problems. Blood pressure tends to go up and down, even in people who have normal blood pressure. If your numbers stay above normal most of the time, you're at risk.

Categories for Blood Pressure Levels in Adults (in mmHg, or millimeters of mercury)

All levels above 120/80 mmHg raise your risk, and the risk grows as blood pressure levels rise. "Prehypertension" means you're likely to end up with HBP, unless you take steps to prevent it.

If you're being treated for HBP and have repeat readings in the normal range, your blood pressure is under control. However, you still have the condition. You should see your doctor and stay on treatment to keep your blood pressure under control.

BLOOD PRESSURE LEVELS			
CATEGORY	**SYSTOLIC (top number)**		**DIASTOLIC (bottom number)**
Normal	Less than 120	And	Less than 80
Prehypertension	120-139	Or	80-89
High Blood Pressure Stage 1	140-159	Or	90-99
High Blood Pressure Stage 2	160 or higher	Or	100 or higher

The ranges in the table apply to most adults (aged 18 and older) who don't have short-term serious illnesses.

Your systolic and diastolic numbers may not be in the same blood pressure category. In this case, the more severe category is the one you're in. For example, if your systolic number is 160 and your diastolic number is 80, you have stage 2 HBP. If your systolic number is 120 and your diastolic number is 95, you have stage 1 HBP.

If you have diabetes or chronic kidney disease, HBP is defined as 130/80 mmHg or higher. HBP numbers also differ for children and teens.

Outlook

Blood pressure tends to rise with age. Following a healthy lifestyle helps some people delay or prevent this rise in blood pressure.

People who have HBP can take steps to control it and reduce their risks for related health problems. Key steps include following a healthy lifestyle, having ongoing medical care, and following the treatment plan that your doctor prescribes.

What Are Overweight and Obesity?

The terms "overweight" and "obesity" refer to a person's overall body weight and where the extra weight comes from. Overweight is having extra body weight from muscle, bone, fat, and/or water. Obesity is having a high amount of extra body fat. The most useful measure of overweight and obesity is the body mass index (BMI). BMI is based on height and weight and is used for adults, children, and teens

Millions of Americans and people worldwide are overweight or obese. Being overweight or obese puts you at risk for many diseases and conditions. The more body fat that you carry around and the more you weigh, the more likely you are to develop heart disease, high blood pressure, type 2 diabetes, gallstones, breathing problems, and certain cancers.

A person's weight is a result of many factors. These factors include environment, family history and genetics, metabolism (the way your body changes food and oxygen into energy), behavior or habits, and other factors.

Certain things, like family history, can't be changed. However, other things—like a person's lifestyle habits—can be changed. You can help prevent or treat overweight and obesity if you:

- Follow a healthful diet, while keeping your calorie needs in mind

- Are physically active

- Limit the time you spend being physically inactive

- Weight loss medicines and surgery also are options for some people who need to lose weight if lifestyle changes don't work.

Outlook

Reaching and staying at a healthy weight is a long-term challenge for people who are overweight or obese. But it also can be a chance to lower your risk of other serious health problems. With the right treatment and motivation, it's possible to lose weight and lower your long-term disease risk.

How Are Overweight and Obesity Diagnosed?

The most common way to find out whether you're overweight or obese is to figure out your body mass index (BMI). BMI is an estimate of body fat and a good gauge of your risk for diseases that occur with more body fat. The higher your BMI, the higher your risk of disease. BMI is calculated from your height and weight. You or your health care provider can use the chart on the following pages, or the National Heart, Lung, and Blood Institute's online BMI calculator to figure out your BMI.

* Weight is measured with underwear but no shoes.

Use the tables on the following two pages to learn your BMI.

- ≈ First, find your height (in inches) on the far left-hand column.

- ≈ Next, move across the row to find your weight (in pounds).

- ≈ Once you've found your weight, move to the very top of that column.

- ≈ This number is your BMI.

Use these tables to learn your Body Mass Index (BMI).
* Weight is measured with underwear but no shoes.

Table 1 - Body Mass Index Table

	Normal						Overweight					Obese					
BMI	**19**	**20**	**21**	**22**	**23**	**24**	**25**	**26**	**27**	**28**	**29**	**30**	**31**	**32**	**33**	**34**	**35**
Height (inches)	Body Weight (pounds)																
58	91	96	100	105	110	115	119	124	129	134	138	143	148	153	158	162	167
59	94	99	104	109	114	119	124	128	133	138	143	148	153	158	163	168	173
60	97	102	107	112	118	123	128	133	138	143	148	153	158	163	168	174	179
61	100	106	111	116	122	127	132	137	143	148	153	158	164	169	174	180	185
62	104	109	115	120	126	131	136	142	147	153	158	164	169	175	180	186	191
63	107	113	118	124	130	135	141	146	152	158	163	169	175	180	186	191	197
64	110	116	122	128	134	140	145	151	157	163	169	174	180	186	192	197	204
65	114	120	126	132	138	144	150	156	162	168	174	180	186	192	198	204	210
66	118	124	130	136	142	148	155	161	167	173	179	186	192	198	204	210	216
67	121	127	134	140	146	153	159	166	172	178	185	191	198	204	211	217	223
68	125	131	138	144	151	158	164	171	177	184	190	197	203	210	216	223	230
69	128	135	142	149	155	162	169	176	182	189	196	203	209	216	223	230	236
70	132	139	146	153	160	167	174	181	188	195	202	209	216	222	229	236	243
71	136	143	150	157	165	172	179	186	193	200	208	215	222	229	236	243	250
72	140	147	154	162	169	177	184	191	199	206	213	221	228	235	242	250	258
73	144	151	159	166	174	182	189	197	204	212	219	227	235	242	250	257	265
74	148	155	163	171	179	186	194	202	210	218	225	233	241	249	256	264	272
75	152	160	168	176	184	192	200	208	216	224	232	240	248	256	264	272	279
76	156	164	172	180	189	197	205	213	221	230	238	246	254	263	271	279	287

For Body Mass Index (BMI) Greater than 35, Go to Table 2

1) First, find your height (in inches) on the far left-hand column.
2) Next, move across the row to find your weight (in pounds).

3) Once you've found your weight, move to the very top of that column.
4) This number is your BMI.

Table 2 - Body Mass Index Table

Height (inches)	Obese				Extreme Obesity														
BMI	36	37	38	39	40	41	42	43	44	45	46	47	48	49	50	51	52	53	54
					Body Weight (pounds)														
58	172	177	181	186	191	196	201	205	210	215	220	224	229	234	239	244	248	253	258
59	178	183	188	193	198	203	208	212	217	222	227	232	237	242	247	252	257	262	267
60	184	189	194	199	204	209	215	220	225	230	235	240	245	250	255	261	266	271	276
61	190	195	201	206	211	217	222	227	232	238	243	248	254	259	264	269	275	280	285
62	196	202	207	213	218	224	229	235	240	246	251	256	262	267	273	278	284	289	295
63	203	208	214	220	225	231	237	242	248	254	259	265	270	278	282	287	293	299	304
64	209	214	221	227	232	238	244	250	256	262	267	273	279	285	291	296	302	308	314
65	216	222	228	234	240	246	252	258	264	270	276	282	288	294	300	306	312	318	324
66	223	229	235	241	247	253	260	266	272	278	284	291	297	303	309	315	322	328	334
67	230	236	242	249	255	261	268	274	280	287	293	299	306	312	319	325	331	338	344
68	236	243	249	256	262	269	276	282	289	295	302	308	315	322	328	335	341	348	354
69	243	250	257	263	270	277	284	291	297	304	311	318	324	331	338	345	351	358	365
70	250	257	264	271	278	285	292	299	306	313	320	327	334	341	348	355	362	369	376
71	257	265	272	279	286	293	301	308	315	322	329	338	343	351	358	365	372	379	386
72	265	272	279	287	294	302	309	316	324	331	338	346	353	361	368	375	383	390	397
73	272	280	288	295	302	310	318	325	333	340	348	355	363	371	378	386	393	401	408
74	280	287	295	303	311	319	326	334	342	350	358	365	373	381	389	396	404	412	420
75	287	295	303	311	319	327	335	343	351	359	367	375	383	391	399	407	415	423	431
76	295	304	312	320	328	336	344	353	361	369	377	385	394	402	410	418	426	435	443

BMI Tables frrom NIH web site

What Does Body Mass Index Mean?

BODY MASS INDEX (BMI)	
18.5 - 24.9	Normal weight
25.0 - 29.9	Overweight
30.0 - 39.9	Obese
40.0 and above	Extreme obesity

ALTHOUGH BMI CAN BE USED FOR MOST MEN AND WOMEN, IT DOES HAVE SOME LIMITS:
It may overestimate body fat in athletes and others who have a muscular build.
It may underestimate body fat in older persons and others who have lost muscle.

What Causes Overweight and Obesity?

Energy Balance

For most people, overweight and obesity are caused by not having energy balance. Weight is balanced by the amount of energy or calories you get from food and drinks (this is called energy IN) equaling the energy your body uses for things like breathing, digesting, and being physically active (this is called energy OUT). Energy balance means that your energy IN equals your energy OUT. To maintain a healthy weight, your energy IN and OUT don't have to balance exactly every day.

IT'S THE BALANCE OVER TIME **THAT HELPS YOU MAINTAIN A HEALTHY WEIGHT**
The same amount of energy IN and energy OUT over time = weight stays the same
More IN than OUT over time = weight gain
More OUT than IN over time = weight loss
Overweight and obesity happen over time when you take in more calories than you use.

Other Causes:

Physical Inactivity

Many Americans aren't very physically active. There are many reasons for this. One reason is that many people spend hours in front of TVs and computers doing work, schoolwork, and leisure activities. In fact, more than 2 hours a day of regular TV viewing time has been linked to overweight and obesity.

Other reasons for not being active include: relying on cars instead of walking to places, fewer physical demands at work or at home because modern technology and conveniences reduce the need to burn calories, and lack of physical education classes in schools for children.

People who are inactive are more likely to gain weight because they don't burn up the calories that they take in from food and drinks. An inactive lifestyle also raises your risk for heart disease, high blood pressure, diabetes, colon cancer, and other health problems.

Environment

Our environment doesn't always help with healthy lifestyle habits; in fact, it encourages obesity. Some reasons include:

ENVIRONMENTAL ISSUES THAT ENCOURAGE OBESITY
Lack of neighborhood sidewalks and safe places for recreation. Not having area parks, trails, sidewalks, and affordable gyms makes it hard for people to be physically active.
Work schedules. People often say that they don't have time to be physically active given the long hours at work and the time spent commuting back and forth to work.
Oversized food portions. Americans are surrounded by huge food portions in restaurants, fast food places, gas stations, movie theaters, supermarkets, and even home. Some of these meals and snacks can feed two or more people. Eating large portions means too much energy IN. Over time, this will cause weight gain if it isn't balanced with physical activity.
Lack of access to healthy foods. Some people don't live in neighborhoods that have supermarkets that sell healthy foods such as fresh fruits and vegetables. Or if they do, these items are often too costly.
Food advertising. Americans are surrounded by ads from food companies. Often children are the targets of advertising for high-calorie, high-fat snacks and sugary drinks. The goal of these ads is to sway people to buy these high-calorie foods, and often they do.

Genes and Family History

Studies of identical twins who have been raised apart show that genes have a strong influence on one's weight. Overweight and obesity tend to run in families. Your chances of being overweight are greater if one or both of your parents are overweight or obese. Your genes also may affect the amount of fat you store in your body and where on your body you carry the extra fat.

Because families also share food and physical activity habits, there is a link between genes and the environment. Children adopt the habits of their parents.

So, a child with overweight parents who eat high-calorie foods and are inactive will likely become overweight like the parents. On the other hand, if a family adopts healthful food and physical activity habits, the child's chance of being overweight or obese is reduced.

Health Conditions

Sometimes hormone problems cause overweight and obesity.
These problems include:

HORMONAL ISSUES THAT CAN CAUSE OVERWEIGHT AND OBE-SITY
Underactive thyroid (also called hypothyroidism). This is a condition in which the thyroid gland doesn't make enough thyroid hormone. Lack of thyroid hormone will slow down your metabolism and cause weight gain. You'll also feel tired and weak.
Cushing's syndrome. This is a condition in which the body's adrenal glands make too much of the hormone cortisol. Cushing's syndrome also can happen when people take high levels of medicines such as prednisone for long periods of time. People with Cushing's syndrome gain weight, have upper-body obesity, a rounded face, fat around the neck, and thin arms and legs.
Polycystic ovarian syndrome (PCOS). This is a condition that affects about 5 to 10 percent of women of childbearing age. Women with PCOS often are obese, have excess hair growth, and have reproductive and other health problems due to high levels of hormones called androgens.

Medicines

Certain medicines such as corticosteroids (for example, prednisone), anti-depressants (for example, Elavil®), and medicines for seizures (for example, Neurontin®) may cause you to gain weight. These medicines can slow the rate at which your body burns calories, increase your appetite, or cause your body to hold on to extra water – all of which can lead to weight gain.

Emotional Factors

Some people eat more than usual when they are bored, angry, or stressed. Over time, overeating will lead to weight gain and may cause overweight or obesity.

Smoking

Some people gain weight when they stop smoking. One reason is that food often tastes and smells better. Another reason is because nicotine raises the rate at which your body burns calories, so you burn fewer calories when you stop smoking. However, smoking is a serious health risk, and quitting is more important than possible weight gain.

Age

As you get older, you tend to lose muscle, especially if you're less active. Muscle loss can slow down the rate at which your body burns calories. If you don't reduce your calorie intake as you get older, you may gain weight. Midlife weight gain in women is mainly due to aging and lifestyle, but menopause also plays a role. Many women gain around 5 pounds during menopause and have more fat around the waist than they did before.

Pregnancy

During pregnancy, women gain weight so that the baby gets proper nourishment and develops normally. After giving birth, some women find it hard to lose the weight. This may lead to overweight or obesity, especially after a few pregnancies.

Lack of Sleep

Studies find that the less people sleep, the more likely they are to be overweight or obese. People who report sleeping 5 hours a night, for example, are much more likely to become obese compared to people who sleep 7-8 hours a night.

People who sleep fewer hours also seem to prefer eating foods that are higher in calories and carbohydrates, which can lead to overeating, weight gain, and obesity over time. Hormones that are released during sleep control appetite and the body's use of energy. For example, insulin controls the rise and fall of blood sugar levels during sleep. People who don't get enough sleep have insulin and blood sugar levels that are similar to those in people who are likely to have diabetes.

Also, people who don't get enough sleep on a regular basis seem to have high levels of a hormone called ghrelin (which causes hunger) and low levels of a hormone called leptin (which normally helps to curb hunger).

Your Pulse and Your Target Heart Rate

Your pulse is your heart rate, or the number of times your heart beats in one minute. Pulse rates vary from person to person. Your pulse is lower when you are at rest and increases when you exercise (because more oxygen-rich blood is needed by the body when you exercise).

Knowing how to take your pulse can help you evaluate your exercise program.

WHAT IS A NORMAL PULSE?	
Age Group	**Normal Heart Rate at Rest**
Children (ages 6-15)	70-100 beats per minute
Adults (age 18 and over)	60-100 beats per minute

How to take your pulse:

 Place the tips of your index, second, and third fingers on the palm side of your other wrist, below the base of the thumb. Or, place the tips of your index and second fingers on your lower neck, on either side of your windpipe.

 Press lightly with your fingers until you feel the blood pulsing beneath your fingers. You might need to move your fingers around slightly up or down until you feel the pulsing.

 Use a watch with a second hand, or look at a clock with a second hand.

 Count the beats you feel for 10 seconds. Multiply this number by six to get your heart rate (pulse) per minute.

Check your pulse: _____ x 6 = _____

(beats in 10 seconds)   (your pulse)

What is maximum heart rate?

The maximum heart rate is the highest your pulse rate can get.

To calculate your predicted maximum heart rate, use this formula:

220 – _____ = _____

(Your Age)   (Predicted Maximum Heart Rate)

Example: a 40-year-old's predicted maximum heart rate is 180.

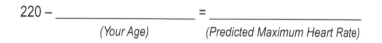

220 – _____40_____ = _____180_____

(Age of 40 Year Old Woman)   (Predicted Maximum Heart Rate)

Your actual maximum heart rate can be determined by a graded exercise test.

Please note that some medicines and medical conditions might affect your maximum heart rate. If you are taking medicines or have a medical condition (such as heart disease, high blood pressure, or diabetes), always ask your doctor if your maximum heart rate/target heart rate will be affected. If so, your heart rate ranges for exercise should be prescribed by your doctor or an exercise specialist.

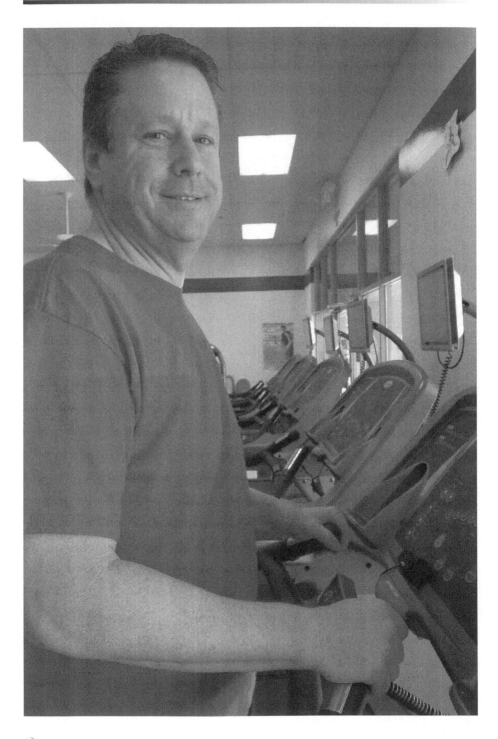

Target heart rate

You gain the most benefits and lessen the risks when you exercise in your target heart rate zone. Usually this is when your exercise heart rate (pulse) is 60 percent to 80 percent of your maximum heart rate. In some cases, your health care provider might decrease your target heart rate zone to begin with 50 percent.

Do not exercise above 85 percent of your maximum heart rate. This increases both cardiovascular and orthopaedic risk and does not add any extra benefit.

> *Always check with your doctor or health care provider before starting an exercise program. You need to know that it is OK to start working out. Your health care provider can help you find a program and target heart rate zone that match your needs, goals, and physical condition.*

When beginning an exercise program, you will need to gradually build up to a level that is within your target heart rate zone, especially if you have not exercised regularly before. Start slowly. Don't push it. Remember we all have to start somewhere. If the exercise feels too hard, slow down. You will reduce your risk of injury and enjoy the exercise more if you don't try to over-do it.

To find out if you are exercising in your target zone (between 60 percent and 80 percent of your maximum heart rate), stop exercising and check your 10-second pulse. A pulse watch is a great thing if you are not exercising on a machine that has the pulse meters built in. I found it to be a good tool when I exercised. A lot of the newer machines at any gym have pulse rate monitors built into the handgrips. If your pulse is below your target zone (see the chart below), increase your rate of exercise. If your pulse is above your target zone, decrease your rate of exercise.

The table (*below*) shows estimated target heart rates for different ages. Look for the age category closest to yours and then read across to find your target heart rate.

Target Heart Rate		
Age	**Target HR Zone 50–85 %**	**Average Maximum Heart Rate 100 %**
20 years	100–170 beats per minute	200 beats per minute
25 years	98–166 beats per minute	195 beats per minute
30 years	95–162 beats per minute	190 beats per minute
35 years	93–157 beats per minute	185 beats per minute
40 years	90–153 beats per minute	180 beats per minute
45 years	88–149 beats per minute	175 beats per minute
50 years	85–145 beats per minute	170 beats per minute
55 years	83–140 beats per minute	165 beats per minute
60 years	80–136 beats per minute	160 beats per minute
65 years	78–132 beats per minute	155 beats per minute
70 years	75–128 beats per minute	150 beats per minute

Your maximum heart rate is about 220 minus your age. The figures above are averages, so use them as general guidelines.

Note: A few high blood pressure medications lower the maximum heart rate and thus the target zone rate. If you're taking such medicine, talk to your doctor to find out if you need to use a lower target heart rate.

Tobacco Facts

Tobacco is one of the strongest cancer-causing agents. Tobacco use is associated with a number of different cancers, including lung cancer, as well as with chronic lung diseases and cardiovascular diseases.

Cigarette smoking remains the leading preventable cause of death in the United States, causing an estimated 438,000 deaths — or about 1 out of every 5 — each year.

In the United States, approximately 38,000 deaths each year are caused by exposure to secondhand smoke.

Lung cancer is the leading cause of cancer death among both men and women in the United States, with 90 percent of lung cancer deaths among men and approximately 80 percent of lung cancer deaths among women attributed to smoking.

Smoking also increases the risk of many other types of cancer, including cancers of the throat, mouth, pancreas, kidney, bladder, and cervix.

People who smoke are up to six times more likely to suffer a heart attack than nonsmokers, and the risk increases with the number of cigarettes smoked. Smoking also causes most cases of chronic obstructive lung disease, which includes bronchitis and emphysema.

In 2007, approximately 19.8 percent of U.S. adults were cigarette smokers.

Twenty-three percent of high school students and 8 percent of middle school students in this country are current cigarette smokers.

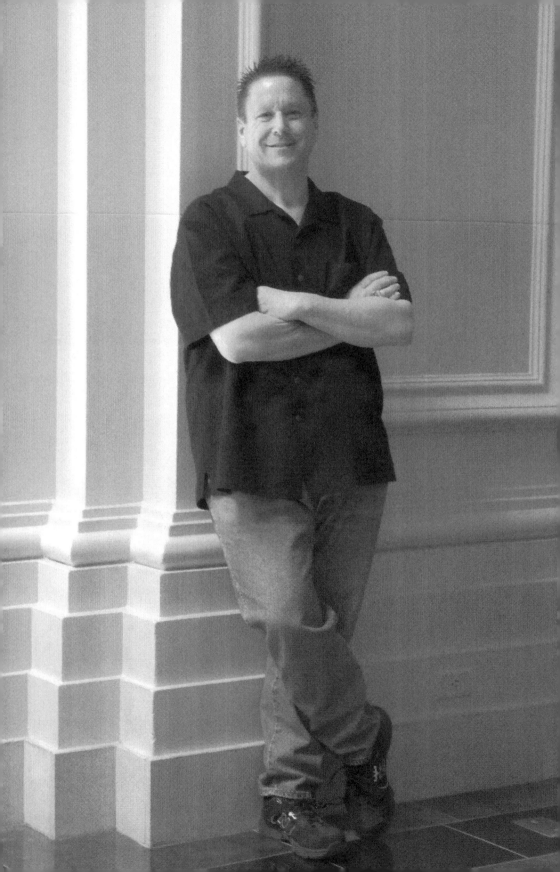

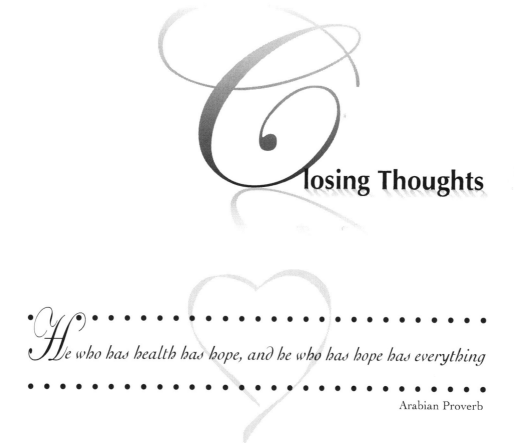

Closing Thoughts

He who has health has hope, and he who has hope has everything

Arabian Proverb

I've had some extraordinary medical challenges in the past couple of years. I never knew I could handle so much. It has been an amazing journey, and I have felt a great sense of accomplishment.

I did not expect to have these problems, nor was I prepared for them, and many people would be quick to say "I told you so." I have tried to deal with them the best that I can. I wish I had a crystal ball to see what the future will bring. In life we may not have a crystal ball, but we have the next best thing, and that is the ability to make a difference in our own lives and change the things we can. I know that by taking action and changing many of my old habits and working on them each day, every day, I am a better person both physically and spiritually. I never take for granted that I got a second chance. Each day I try to be a better person than I was the day before. It is so important that each of us participate in our own well-being every day.

Schedule that checkup. Talk to your doctor. Start walking. Do something today that you didn't do yesterday to promote your own physical fitness and health.

If you do this,

you will accomplish things

and dreams you never

knew existed!

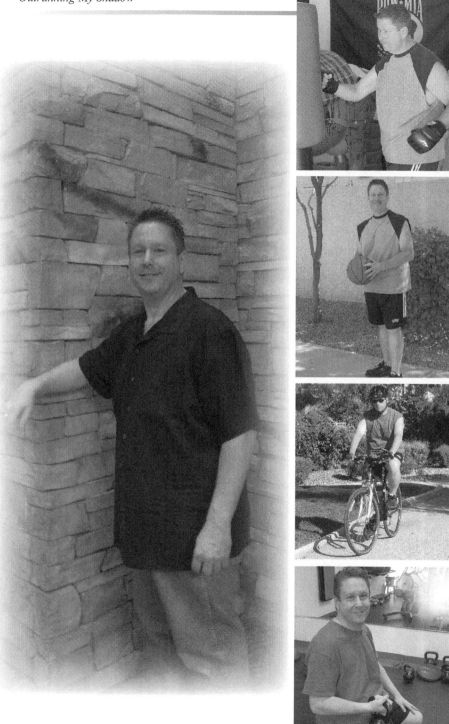

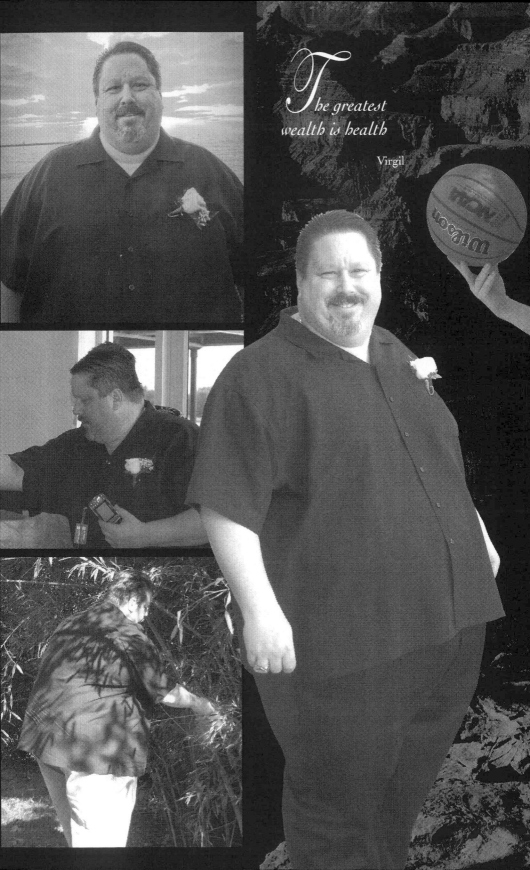

The greatest
wealth is health

Virgil

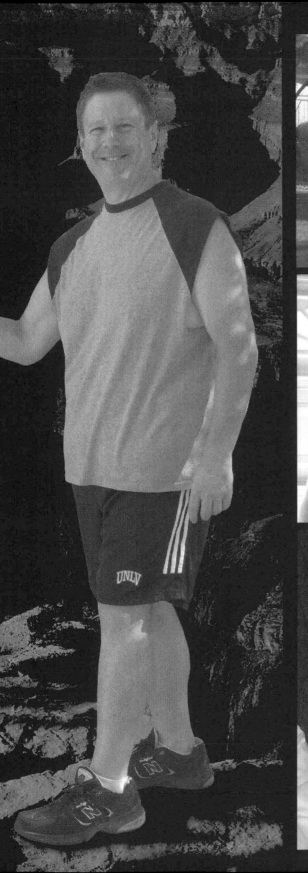
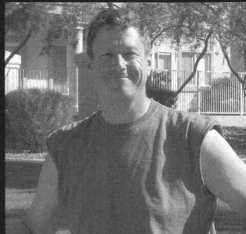
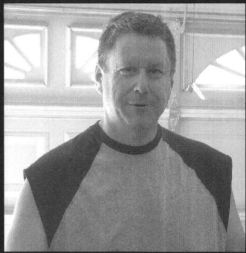
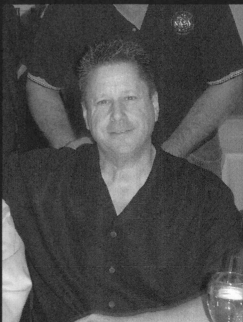

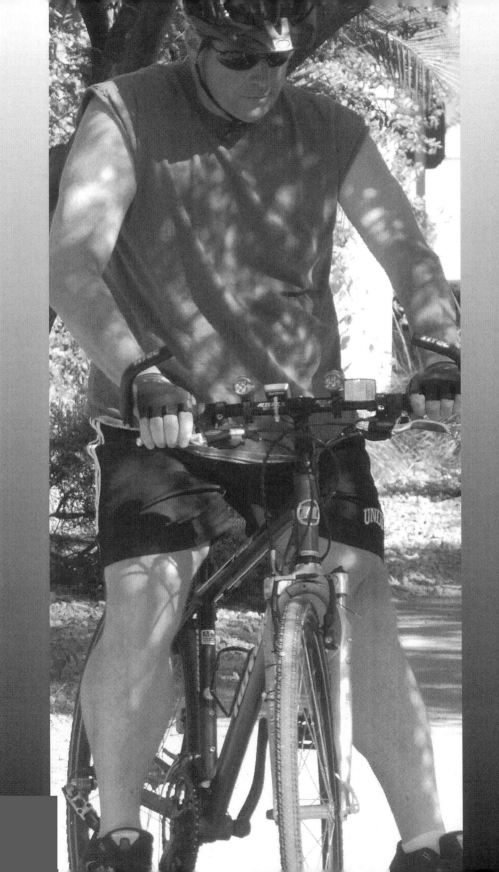

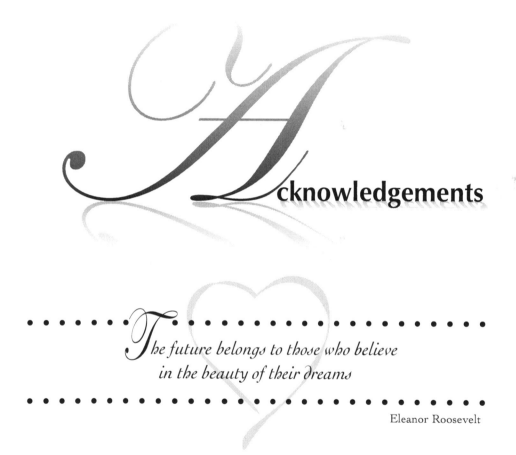

Acknowledgements

*The future belongs to those who believe
in the beauty of their dreams*

Eleanor Roosevelt

A special thanks

and heartfelt appreciation

to a few of the many people

who have helped me . . .

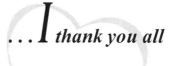

...I thank you all

from the bottom

of my heart!

Dr. Eric Wikler, D.O.

Dr. Leo J. Spaccavento, M.D., F.A.C.C.

Dr. V.C. Smith, M.D., F.A.C.C.

Dr. Glen A. Hirsch, M.D.

Dr. Hanna DeMarco, M.D.

The Cleveland Clinic Cardiology Department and Coronary Care Unit

The Registered Nurses and Exercise Physiologists
at the Cardio Pulmonary Rehabilitation Unit of St. Rose Dominican Hospital,
Jackie, Kathy, Emily and Keri

My co-workers who always listened, cared, supported and encouraged me

Bradley Howatt, Jimmy Lee, James Williams, Glen Stephens

Of course all my family and friends

Double special thanks to my sister Candy
who made the best fresh chicken soup
and kept me focused when things seemed too much for me to handle

Notes